THE YOGA OF DIVINE WORKS

THE SYNTHESIS OF YOGA

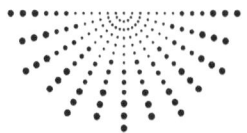

SRI AUROBINDO

CONTENTS

INTRODUCTION

Chapter I. Life and Yoga	3
Chapter II. The Three Steps of Nature	7
Chapter III. The Threefold Life	15
Chapter IV. The Systems of Yoga	24
Chapter V. The Synthesis of the Systems	32

THE YOGA OF DIVINE WORKS

Chapter I. The Four Aids	43
Chapter II. Self-Consecration	55
Chapter III. Self-Surrender in Works — The Way of the Gita	70
Chapter IV. The Sacrifice, the Triune Path and the Lord of the Sacrifice	83
Chapter V. The Ascent of the Sacrifice–1	104
Chapter VI. The Ascent of the Sacrifice–2	122
Chapter VII. Standards of Conduct and Spiritual Freedom	145
Chapter VIII. The Supreme Will	160
Chapter IX. Equality and the Annihilation of Ego	170
Chapter X. The Three Modes of Nature	179
Chapter XI. The Master of the Work	188
Chapter XII. The Divine Work	204
Also by SRI AUROBINDO	215

INTRODUCTION

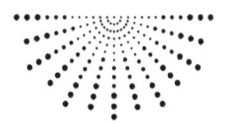

CHAPTER I. LIFE AND YOGA

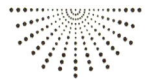

THERE are two necessities of Nature's workings which seem always to intervene in the greater forms of human activity, whether these belong to our ordinary fields of movement or seek those exceptional spheres and fulfilments which appear to us high and divine. Every such form tends towards a harmonised complexity and totality which again breaks apart into various channels of special effort and tendency, only to unite once more in a larger and more puissant synthesis. Secondly, development into forms is an imperative rule of effective manifestation; yet all truth and practice too strictly formulated becomes old and loses much, if not all, of its virtue; it must be constantly renovated by fresh streams of the spirit revivifying the dead or dying vehicle and changing it, if it is to acquire a new life. To be perpetually reborn is the condition of a material immortality. We are in an age, full of the throes of travail, when all forms of thought and activity that have in themselves any strong power of utility or any secret virtue of persistence are being subjected to a supreme test and given their opportunity of rebirth. The world today presents the aspect of a huge cauldron of Medea in which all things are being cast, shredded into pieces, experimented on, combined and recombined either to perish and provide the scattered material of new forms or to emerge rejuvenated and changed for a fresh term of existence. Indian Yoga, in its essence a special action or formulation of certain great powers of Nature, itself specialised, divided and variously formulated, is potentially one of these dynamic elements of the future life of humanity. The child of immemorial ages, preserved by its vitality and truth into our modern times, it is now emerging from the secret schools and ascetic retreats in which it had taken refuge and is seeking its place in the future sum of living human powers and utilities. But it has first to rediscover itself, bring to the surface the profoundest reason of its being in that general truth and that unceasing aim of Nature which it represents, and find by virtue of this new self-knowledge and self-appreciation its own recovered and larger synthesis. Reorganising itself, it will enter more easily and powerfully into the reorganised life of the race which its processes claim to lead within into the most secret penetralia and upward to the highest altitudes of existence and personality.

In the right view both of life and of Yoga all life is either consciously or subconsciously a Yoga. For we mean by this term a methodised effort towards self-perfection by the expression of the secret potentialities latent in the being and—highest condition of victory in that effort—a union of the human individual with the universal and transcendent Existence we see partially expressed in man and in the Cosmos. But all life, when we look behind its appearances, is a vast Yoga of Nature who attempts in the conscious and the subconscious to realise her perfection in an ever-increasing expression of her yet unrealised potentialities and to unite herself with her own divine reality. In man, her thinker, she for the first time upon this Earth devises self-conscious means and willed arrangements of activity by which this great purpose may be more swiftly and puissantly attained. Yoga, as Swami Vivekananda has said, may be regarded as a means of compressing one's evolution into a single life or a few years or even a few months of bodily existence. A given system of Yoga, then, can be no more than a selection or a compression, into narrower but more energetic forms of intensity, of the general methods which are already being used loosely, largely, in a leisurely movement, with a profuser apparent waste of material and energy but with a more complete combination by the great Mother in her vast upward labour. It is this view of Yoga that can alone form the basis for a sound and rational synthesis of Yogic methods. For then Yoga ceases to appear something mystic and abnormal which has no relation to the ordinary processes of the World-Energy or the purpose she keeps in view in her two great movements of subjective and objective self-fulfilment; it reveals itself rather as an intense and exceptional use of powers that she has already manifested or is progressively organising in her less exalted but more general operations. Yogic methods have something of the same relation to the customary psychological workings of man as has the scientific handling of the force of electricity or of steam to their normal operations in Nature. And they, too, like the operations of Science, are formed upon a knowledge developed and confirmed by regular experiment, practical analysis and constant result. All Rajayoga, for instance, depends on this perception and experience that our inner elements, combinations, functions, forces, can be separated or dissolved, can be new-combined and set to novel and formerly impossible workings or can be transformed and resolved into a new general synthesis by fixed internal processes. Hathayoga similarly depends on this perception and experience that the vital forces and functions to which our life is normally subjected and whose ordinary operations seem set and indispensable, can be mastered and the operations changed or suspended with results that would otherwise be impossible and that seem miraculous to those who have not seized the rationale of their process. And if in some other of its forms this character of Yoga is less apparent, because they are more intuitive and less mechanical, nearer, like the Yoga of Devotion, to a supernal ecstasy or, like the Yoga of Knowledge, to a supernal infinity of consciousness and being, yet they too start from the use of some principal faculty in us by ways and for ends not contemplated in its everyday spontaneous workings. All methods grouped under the common name of Yoga are special psychological processes founded on a fixed truth of Nature and developing, out of normal functions, powers and results which were always latent but which her ordinary movements do not easily or do not often manifest.

But as in physical knowledge the multiplication of scientific processes has its disadvantages, as that tends, for instance, to develop a victorious artificiality which overwhelms our natural human life under a load of machinery and to purchase certain forms of freedom and mastery at the price of an increased servitude, so the preoccupation with Yogic processes and their exceptional results may have its disadvantages and losses. The Yogin tends to draw away from the common existence and lose his hold upon it; he tends to purchase wealth of spirit by an impoverishment of his human activities, the inner freedom by an outer death. If he gains God, he loses life, or if he turns his efforts outward to conquer life, he is in danger of losing God. Therefore we see in India that a sharp incompatibility has been created between life in the world and spiritual growth and perfection, and although the tradition and ideal of a victorious harmony between the inner attraction and the outer demand remains, it is little or else very imperfectly exemplified. In fact, when a man turns his vision and energy inward and enters on the path of Yoga, he is popularly supposed to be lost inevitably to the great stream of our collective existence and the secular effort of humanity. So strongly has the idea prevailed, so much has it been emphasised by prevalent philosophies and religions that to escape from life is now commonly considered as not only the necessary condition, but the general object of Yoga. No synthesis of Yoga can be satisfying which does not, in its aim, reunite God and Nature in a liberated and perfected human life or, in its method, not only permit but favour the harmony of our inner and outer activities and experiences in the divine consummation of both. For man is precisely that term and symbol of a higher Existence descended into the material world in which it is possible for the lower to transfigure itself and put on the nature of the higher and the higher to reveal itself in the forms of the lower. To avoid the life which is given him for the realisation of that possibility, can never be either the indispensable condition or the whole and ultimate object of his supreme endeavour or of his most powerful means of self-fulfilment. It can only be a temporary necessity under certain conditions or a specialised extreme effort imposed on the individual so as to prepare a greater general possibility for the race. The true and full object and utility of Yoga can only be accomplished when the conscious Yoga in man becomes, like the subconscious Yoga in Nature, outwardly conterminous with life itself and we can once more, looking out both on the path and the achievement, say in a more perfect and luminous sense:

"All life is Yoga."

CHAPTER II. THE THREE STEPS OF NATURE

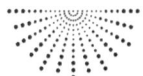

WE RECOGNISE then, in the past developments of Yoga, a specialising and separative tendency which, like all things in Nature, had its justifying and even imperative utility and we seek a synthesis of the specialised aims and methods which have, in consequence, come into being. But in order that we may be wisely guided in our effort, we must know, first, the general principle and purpose underlying this separative impulse and, next, the particular utilities upon which the method of each school of Yoga is founded. For the general principle we must interrogate the universal workings of Nature herself, recognising in her no merely specious and illusive activity of a distorting Maya, but the cosmic energy and working of God Himself in His universal being formulating and inspired by a vast, an infinite and yet a minutely selective Wisdom, *prajñā prasṛtā purāṇī* of the Upanishad, Wisdom that went forth from the Eternal since the beginning. For the particular utilities we must cast a penetrative eye on the different methods of Yoga and distinguish among the mass of their details the governing idea which they serve and the radical force which gives birth and energy to their processes of effectuation. Afterwards we may more easily find the one common principle and the one common power from which all derive their being and tendency, towards which all subconsciously move and in which, therefore, it is possible for all consciously to unite.

The progressive self-manifestation of Nature in man, termed in modern language his evolution, must necessarily depend upon three successive elements. There is that which is already evolved; there is that which, still imperfect, still partly fluid, is persistently in the stage of conscious evolution; and there is that which is to be evolved and may perhaps be already displayed, if not constantly, then occasionally or with some regularity of recurrence, in primary formations or in others more developed and, it may well be, even in some, however rare, that are near to the highest possible realisation of our present humanity. For the march of Nature is not drilled to a regular and mechanical forward stepping. She reaches constantly beyond herself even at the cost of subsequent deplorable retreats. She has rushes; she has splendid and mighty outbursts; she has immense realisations. She storms sometimes passionately forward hoping to take the kingdom of heaven by violence. And these self-exceedings are the revelation of that in her which is most divine or else most diabolical, but in either case the most puissant to bring her rapidly forward towards her goal.

That which Nature has evolved for us and has firmly founded is the bodily life. She has effected a certain combination and harmony of the two inferior but most fundamentally necessary elements of our action and progress upon earth,—Matter, which, however the too ethereally spiritual may despise it, is our foundation and the first condition of all our energies and realisations, and the Life-Energy which is our means of existence in a material body and the basis there even of our mental and spiritual activities. She has successfully achieved a certain stability of her constant material movement which is at once sufficiently steady and durable and sufficiently pliable and mutable to provide a fit dwelling-place and instrument for the progressively manifesting god in humanity. This is what is meant by the fable in the Aitareya Upanishad which tells us that the gods rejected the animal forms successively offered to them by the Divine Self and only when man was produced, cried out, "This indeed is perfectly made," and consented to enter in. She has effected also a working compromise between the inertia of matter and the active Life that lives in and feeds on it, by which not only is vital existence sustained, but the fullest developments of mentality are rendered possible. This equilibrium constitutes the basic status of Nature in man and is termed in the language of Yoga his gross body composed of the material or food sheath and the nervous system or vital vehicle.[1]

If, then, this inferior equilibrium is the basis and first means of the higher movements which the universal Power contemplates and if it constitutes the vehicle in which the Divine here seeks to reveal Itself, if the Indian saying is true that the body is the instrument provided for the fulfilment of the right law of our nature, then any final recoil from the physical life must be a turning away from the completeness of the divine Wisdom and a renunciation of its aim in earthly manifestation. Such a refusal may be, owing to some secret law of their development, the right attitude for certain individuals, but never the aim intended for mankind. It can be, therefore, no integral Yoga which ignores the body or makes its annulment or its rejection indispensable to a perfect spirituality. Rather, the perfecting of the body also should be the last triumph of the Spirit and to make the bodily life also divine must be God's final seal upon His work in the universe. The obstacle which the physical presents to the spiritual is no argument for the rejection of the physical; for in the unseen providence of things our greatest difficulties are our best opportunities. A supreme difficulty is Nature's indication to us of a supreme conquest to be won and an ultimate problem to be solved; it is not a warning of an inextricable snare to be shunned or of an enemy too strong for us from whom we must flee.

Equally, the vital and nervous energies in us are there for a great utility; they too demand the divine realisation of their possibilities in our ultimate fulfilment. The great part assigned to this element in the universal scheme is powerfully emphasised by the catholic wisdom of the Upanishads. "As the spokes of a wheel in its nave, so in the Life-Energy is all established, the triple knowledge and the Sacrifice and the power of the strong and the purity of the wise. Under the control of the LifeEnergy is all this that is established in the triple heaven."[2] It is therefore no integral Yoga that kills these vital energies, forces them into a nerveless quiescence or roots them out as the source of noxious activities. Their purification, not their destruction,—their transformation, control and utilisation is the aim in view with which they have been created and developed in us.

If the bodily life is what Nature has firmly evolved for us as her base and first instrument, it is our mental life that she is evolving as her immediate next aim and superior instrument. This in her ordinary exaltations is the lofty preoccupying thought in her; this, except in her periods of exhaustion and recoil into a reposeful and recuperating obscurity, is her constant pursuit wherever she can get free from the trammels of her first vital and physical realisations. For here in man we have a distinction which is of the utmost importance. He has in him not a single mentality, but a double and a triple, the mind material and nervous, the pure intellectual mind which liberates itself from the illusions of the body and the senses, and a divine mind above intellect which in its turn liberates itself from the imperfect modes of the logically discriminative and imaginative reason. Mind in man is first emmeshed in the life of the body, where in the plant it is entirely involved and in animals always imprisoned. It accepts this life as not only the first but the whole condition of its activities and serves its needs as if they were the entire aim of existence. But the bodily life in man is a base, not the aim, his first condition and not his last determinant. In the just idea of the ancients man is essentially the thinker, the Manu, the mental being who leads the life and the body,[3] not the animal who is led by them. The true human existence, therefore, only begins when the intellectual mentality emerges out of the material and we begin more and more to live in the mind independent of the nervous and physical obsession and in the measure of that liberty are able to accept rightly and rightly to use the life of the body. For freedom and not a skilful subjection is the true means of mastery. A free, not a compulsory acceptance of the conditions, the enlarged and sublimated conditions of our physical being, is the high human ideal. But beyond this intellectual mentality is the divine.

The mental life thus evolving in man is not, indeed, a common possession. In actual appearance it would seem as if it were only developed to the fullest in individuals and as if there were great numbers and even the majority in whom it is either a small and ill-organised part of their normal nature or not evolved at all or latent and not easily made active. Certainly, the mental life is not a finished evolution of Nature; it is not yet firmly founded in the human animal. The sign is that the fine and full equilibrium of vitality and matter, the sane, robust, long-lived human body is ordinarily found only in races or classes of men who reject the effort of thought, its disturbances, its tensions, or think only with the material mind. Civilised man has yet to establish an equilibrium between the fully active mind and the body; he does not normally possess it. Indeed, the increasing effort towards a more intense mental life seems to create, frequently, an increasing disequilibrium of the human elements, so that it is possible for eminent scientists to describe genius as a form of insanity, a result of degeneration, a pathological morbidity of Nature. The phenomena which are used to justify this exaggeration, when taken not separately, but in connection with all other relevant data, point to a different truth. Genius is one attempt of the universal Energy to so quicken and intensify our intellectual powers that they shall be prepared for those more puissant, direct and rapid faculties which constitute the play of the supra-intellectual or divine mind. It is not, then, a freak, an inexplicable phenomenon, but a perfectly natural next step in the right line of her evolution. She has harmonised the bodily life with the material mind, she is harmonising it with the play of the intellectual mentality; for that, although it tends to a depression of the full animal and vital vigour, need not produce active disturbances. And she is shooting yet beyond in the attempt to reach a still higher level. Nor are the disturbances created by her process as great as is often represented. Some of them are the crude beginnings of new manifestations; others are an easily corrected movement of disintegration, often fruitful of fresh activities and always a small price to pay for the far-reaching results that she has in view.

We may perhaps, if we consider all the circumstances, come to this conclusion that mental life, far from being a recent appearance in man, is the swift repetition in him of a previous achievement from which the Energy in the race had undergone one of her deplorable recoils. The savage is perhaps not so much the first forefather of civilised man as the degenerate descendant of a previous civilisation. For if the actuality of intellectual achievement is unevenly distributed, the capacity is spread everywhere. It has been seen that in individual cases even the racial type considered by us the lowest, the negro fresh from the perennial barbarism of Central Africa, is capable, without admixture of blood, without waiting for future generations, of the intellectual culture, if not yet of the intellectual accomplishment of the dominant European. Even in the mass men seem to need, in favourable circumstances, only a few generations to cover ground that ought apparently to be measured in the terms of millenniums. Either, then, man by his privilege as a mental being is exempt from the full burden of the tardy laws of evolution or else he already represents and with helpful conditions and in the right stimulating atmosphere can always display a high level of material capacity for the activities of the intellectual life. It is not mental incapacity, but the long rejection or seclusion from opportunity and withdrawal of the awakening impulse that creates the savage. Barbarism is an intermediate sleep, not an original darkness.

Moreover the whole trend of modern thought and modern endeavour reveals itself to the observant eye as a large conscious effort of Nature in man to effect a general level of intellectual equipment, capacity and farther possibility by universalising the opportunities which modern civilisation affords for the mental life. Even the preoccupation of the European intellect, the protagonist of this tendency, with material Nature and the externalities of existence is a necessary part of the effort. It seeks to prepare a sufficient basis in man's physical being and vital energies and in his material environment for his full mental possibilities. By the spread of education, by the advance of the backward races, by the elevation of depressed classes, by the multiplication of labour-saving appliances, by the movement towards ideal social and economic conditions, by the labour of Science towards an improved health, longevity and sound physique in civilised humanity, the sense and drift of this vast movement translates itself in easily intelligible signs. The right or at least the ultimate means may not always be employed, but their aim is the right preliminary aim,— a sound individual and social body and the satisfaction of the legitimate needs and demands of the material mind, sufficient ease, leisure, equal opportunity, so that the whole of mankind and no longer only the favoured race, class or individual may be free to develop the emotional and intellectual being to its full capacity. At present the material and economic aim may predominate, but always, behind, there works or there waits in reserve the higher and major impulse.

And when the preliminary conditions are satisfied, when the great endeavour has found its base, what will be the nature of that farther possibility which the activities of the intellectual life must serve? If Mind is indeed Nature's highest term, then the entire development of the rational and imaginative intellect and the harmonious satisfaction of the emotions and sensibilities must be to themselves sufficient. But if, on the contrary, man is more than a reasoning and emotional animal, if beyond that which is being evolved, there is something that has to be evolved, then it may well be that the fullness of the mental life, the suppleness, flexibility and wide capacity of the intellect, the ordered richness of emotion and sensibility may be only a passage towards the development of a higher life and of more powerful faculties which are yet to manifest and to take possession of the lower instrument, just as mind itself has so taken possession of the body that the physical being no longer lives only for its own satisfaction but provides the foundation and the materials for a superior activity.

The assertion of a higher than the mental life is the whole foundation of Indian philosophy and its acquisition and organisation is the veritable object served by the methods of Yoga. Mind is not the last term of evolution, not an ultimate aim, but, like body, an instrument. It is even so termed in the language of Yoga, the inner instrument.[4] And Indian tradition asserts that this which is to be manifested is not a new term in human experience, but has been developed before and has even governed humanity in certain periods of its development. In any case, in order to be known it must at one time have been partly developed. And if since then Nature has sunk back from her achievement, the reason must always be found in some unrealised harmony, some insufficiency of the intellectual and material basis to which she has now returned, some over-specialisation of the higher to the detriment of the lower existence.

But what then constitutes this higher or highest existence to which our evolution is tending? In order to answer the question we have to deal with a class of supreme experiences, a class of unusual conceptions which it is difficult to represent accurately in any other language than the ancient Sanskrit tongue in which alone they have been to some extent systematised. The only approximate terms in the English language have other associations and their use may lead to many and even serious inaccuracies. The terminology of Yoga recognises besides the status of our physical and vital being, termed the gross body and doubly composed of the food sheath and the vital vehicle, besides the status of our mental being, termed the subtle body and singly composed of the mind sheath or mental vehicle,[5] a third, supreme and divine status of supra-mental being, termed the causal body and composed of a fourth and a fifth vehicle[6] which are described as those of knowledge and bliss. But this knowledge is not a systematised result of mental questionings and reasonings, not a temporary arrangement of conclusions and opinions in the terms of the highest probability, but rather a pure self-existent and self-luminous Truth. And this bliss is not a supreme pleasure of the heart and sensations with the experience of pain and sorrow as its background, but a delight also self-existent and independent of objects and particular experiences, a self-delight which is the very nature, the very stuff, as it were, of a transcendent and infinite existence.

Do such psychological conceptions correspond to anything real and possible? All Yoga asserts them as its ultimate experience and supreme aim. They form the governing principles of our highest possible state of consciousness, our widest possible range of existence. There is, we say, a harmony of supreme faculties, corresponding roughly to the psychological faculties of revelation, inspiration and intuition, yet acting not in the intuitive reason or the divine mind, but on a still higher plane, which see Truth directly face to face, or rather live in the truth of things both universal and transcendent and are its formulation and luminous activity. And these faculties are the light of a conscious existence superseding the egoistic and itself both cosmic and transcendent, the nature of which is Bliss. These are obviously divine and, as man is at present apparently constituted, superhuman states of consciousness and activity. A trinity of transcendent existence, self-awareness and self-delight[7] is, indeed, the metaphysical description of the supreme Atman, the self-formulation, to our awakened knowledge, of the Unknowable whether conceived as a pure Impersonality or as a cosmic Personality manifesting the universe. But in Yoga they are regarded also in their psychological aspects as states of subjective existence to which our waking consciousness is now alien, but which dwell in us in a superconscious plane and to which, therefore, we may always ascend.

For, as is indicated by the name, causal body (*kāraṇa*), as opposed to the two others which are instruments (*karaṇa*), this crowning manifestation is also the source and effective power of all that in the actual evolution has preceded it. Our mental activities are, indeed, a derivation, selection and, so long as they are divided from the truth that is secretly their source, a deformation of the divine knowledge. Our sensations and emotions have the same relation to the Bliss, our vital forces and actions to the aspect of Will or Force assumed by the divine consciousness, our physical being to the pure essence of that Bliss and Consciousness. The evolution which we observe and of which we are the terrestrial summit may be considered, in a sense, as an inverse manifestation, by which these supreme Powers in their unity and their diversity use, develop and perfect the imperfect substance and activities of Matter, of Life and of Mind so that they, the inferior modes, may express in mutable relativity an increasing harmony of the divine and eternal states from which they are born. If this be the truth of the universe, then the goal of evolution is also its cause, it is that which is immanent in its elements and out of them is liberated. But the liberation is surely imperfect if it is only an escape and there is no return upon the containing substance and activities to exalt and transform them. The immanence itself would have no credible reason for being if it did not end in such a transfiguration. But if human mind can become capable of the glories of the divine Light, human emotion and sensibility can be transformed into the mould and assume the measure and movement of the supreme Bliss, human action not only represent but feel itself to be the motion of a divine and non-egoistic Force and the physical substance of our being sufficiently partake of the purity of the supernal essence, sufficiently unify plasticity and durable constancy to support and prolong these highest experiences and agencies, then all the long labour of Nature will end in a crowning justification and her evolutions reveal their profound significance.

So dazzling is even a glimpse of this supreme existence and so absorbing its attraction that, once seen, we feel readily justified in neglecting all else for its pursuit. Even, by an opposite exaggeration to that which sees all things in Mind and the mental life as an exclusive ideal, Mind comes to be regarded as an unworthy deformation and a supreme obstacle, the source of an illusory universe, a negation of the Truth and itself to be denied and all its works and results annulled if we desire the final liberation. But this is a half-truth which errs by regarding only the actual limitations of Mind and ignores its divine intention. The ultimate knowledge is that which perceives and accepts God in the universe as well as beyond the universe; the integral Yoga is that which, having found the Transcendent, can return upon the universe and possess it, retaining the power freely to descend as well as ascend the great stair of existence. For if the eternal Wisdom exists at all, the faculty of Mind also must have some high use and destiny. That use must depend on its place in the ascent and in the return and that destiny must be a fulfilment and transfiguration, not a rooting out or an annulling.

We perceive, then, these three steps in Nature, a bodily life which is the basis of our existence here in the material world, a mental life into which we emerge and by which we raise the bodily to higher uses and enlarge it into a greater completeness, and a divine existence which is at once the goal of the other two and returns upon them to liberate them into their highest possibilities. Regarding none of them as either beyond our reach or below our nature and the destruction of none of them as essential to the ultimate attainment, we accept this liberation and fulfilment as part at least and a large and important part of the aim of Yoga.

---

1. *annakoṣa* and *prāṇakoṣa*.
2. Prasna Upanishad II.
3. *manomayaḥ prāṇaśarīranetā*. Mundaka Upanishad II. 2. 8.
4. *antaḥkaraṇa*.
5. *manaḥ-koṣa*.
6. *vijñānakoṣa* and *ānandakoṣa*.
7. *saccidānanda*.

CHAPTER III. THE THREEFOLD LIFE

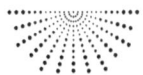

NATURE, then, is an evolution or progressive self-manifestation of an eternal and secret existence, with three successive forms as her three steps of ascent. And we have consequently as the condition of all our activities these three mutually interdependent possibilities, the bodily life, the mental existence and the veiled spiritual being which is in the involution the cause of the others and in the evolution their result. Preserving and perfecting the physical, fulfilling the mental, it is Nature's aim and it should be ours to unveil in the perfected body and mind the transcendent activities of the Spirit. As the mental life does not abrogate but works for the elevation and better utilisation of the bodily existence, so too the spiritual should not abrogate but transfigure our intellectual, emotional, aesthetic and vital activities.

For man, the head of terrestrial Nature, the sole earthly frame in which her full evolution is possible, is a triple birth. He has been given a living frame in which the body is the vessel and life the dynamic means of a divine manifestation. His activity is centred in a progressive mind which aims at perfecting itself as well as the house in which it dwells and the means of life that it uses, and is capable of awaking by a progressive self-realisation to its own true nature as a form of the Spirit. He culminates in what he always really was, the illumined and beatific spirit which is intended at last to irradiate life and mind with its now concealed splendours.

Since this is the plan of the divine Energy in humanity, the whole method and aim of our existence must work by the interaction of these three elements in the being. As a result of their separate formulation in Nature, man has open to him a choice between three kinds of life, the ordinary material existence, a life of mental activity and progress and the unchanging spiritual beatitude. But he can, as he progresses, combine these three forms, resolve their discords into a harmonious rhythm and so create in himself the whole godhead, the perfect Man.

In ordinary Nature they have each their own characteristic and governing impulse.

The characteristic energy of bodily Life is not so much in progress as in persistence, not so much in individual self-enlargement as in self-repetition. There is, indeed, in physical Nature a progression from type to type, from the vegetable to the animal, from the animal to man; for even in inanimate Matter Mind is at work. But once a type is marked off physically, the chief immediate preoccupation of the terrestrial Mother seems to be to keep it in being by a constant reproduction. For Life always seeks immortality; but since individual form is impermanent and only the idea of a form is permanent in the consciousness that creates the universe,—for there it does not perish,—such constant reproduction is the only possible material immortality. Self-preservation, self-repetition, self-multiplication are necessarily, then, the predominant instincts of all material existence. Material life seems ever to move in a fixed cycle.

The characteristic energy of pure Mind is change, and the more our mentality acquires elevation and organisation, the more this law of Mind assumes the aspect of a continual enlargement, improvement and better arrangement of its gains and so of a continual passage from a smaller and simpler to a larger and more complex perfection. For Mind, unlike bodily life, is infinite in its field, elastic in its expansion, easily variable in its formations. Change, then, self-enlargement and self-improvement are its proper instincts. Mind too moves in cycles, but these are ever-enlarging spirals. Its faith is perfectibility, its watchword is progress.

The characteristic law of Spirit is self-existent perfection and immutable infinity. It possesses always and in its own right the immortality which is the aim of Life and the perfection which is the goal of Mind. The attainment of the eternal and the realisation of that which is the same in all things and beyond all things, equally blissful in universe and outside it, untouched by the imperfections and limitations of the forms and activities in which it dwells, are the glory of the spiritual life.

In each of these forms Nature acts both individually and collectively; for the Eternal affirms Himself equally in the single form and in the group-existence, whether family, clan and nation or groupings dependent on less physical principles or the supreme group of all, our collective humanity. Man also may seek his own individual good from any or all of these spheres of activity, or identify himself in them with the collectivity and live for it, or, rising to a truer perception of this complex universe, harmonise the individual realisation with the collective aim. For as it is the right relation of the soul with the Supreme, while it is in the universe, neither to assert egoistically its separate being nor to blot itself out in the Indefinable, but to realise its unity with the Divine and the world and unite them in the individual, so the right relation of the individual with the collectivity is neither to pursue egoistically his own material or mental progress or spiritual salvation without regard to his fellows, nor for the sake of the community to suppress or maim his proper development, but to sum up in himself all its best and completest possibilities and pour them out by thought, action and all other means on his surroundings so that the whole race may approach nearer to the attainment of its supreme personalities.

It follows that the object of the material life must be to fulfil, above all things, the vital aim of Nature. The whole aim of the material man is to live, to pass from birth to death with as much comfort or enjoyment as may be on the way, but anyhow to live. He can subordinate this aim, but only to physical Nature's other instincts, the reproduction of the individual and the conservation of the type in the family, class or community. Self, domesticity, the accustomed order of the society and of the nation are the constituents of the material existence. Its immense importance in the economy of Nature is self-evident, and commensurate is the importance of the human type which represents it. He assures her of the safety of the framework she has made and of the orderly continuance and conservation of her past gains.

But by that very utility such men and the life they lead are condemned to be limited, irrationally conservative and earthbound. The customary routine, the customary institutions, the inherited or habitual forms of thought,—these things are the life-breath of their nostrils. They admit and jealously defend the changes compelled by the progressive mind in the past, but combat with equal zeal the changes that are being made by it in the present. For to the material man the living progressive thinker is an ideologue, dreamer or madman. The old Semites who stoned the living prophets and adored their memories when dead, were the very incarnation of this instinctive and unintelligent principle in Nature. In the ancient Indian distinction between the once born and the twice born, it is to this material man that the former description can be applied. He does Nature's inferior works; he assures the basis for her higher activities; but not to him easily are opened the glories of her second birth.

Yet he admits so much of spirituality as has been enforced on his customary ideas by the great religious outbursts of the past and he makes in his scheme of society a place, venerable though not often effective, for the priest or the learned theologian who can be trusted to provide him with a safe and ordinary spiritual pabulum. But to the man who would assert for himself the liberty of spiritual experience and the spiritual life, he assigns, if he admits him at all, not the vestment of the priest but the robe of the Sannyasin. Outside society let him exercise his dangerous freedom. So he may even serve as a human lightning-rod receiving the electricity of the Spirit and turning it away from the social edifice.

Nevertheless it is possible to make the material man and his life moderately progressive by imprinting on the material mind the custom of progress, the habit of conscious change, the fixed idea of progression as a law of life. The creation by this means of progressive societies in Europe is one of the greatest triumphs of Mind over Matter. But the physical nature has its revenge; for the progress made tends to be of the grosser and more outward kind and its attempts at a higher or a more rapid movement bring about great wearinesses, swift exhaustions, startling recoils.

It is possible also to give the material man and his life a moderate spirituality by accustoming him to regard in a religious spirit all the institutions of life and its customary activities. The creation of such spiritualised communities in the East has been one of the greatest triumphs of Spirit over Matter. Yet here, too, there is a defect; for this often tends only to the creation of a religious temperament, the most outward form of spirituality. Its higher manifestations, even the most splendid and puissant, either merely increase the number of souls drawn out of social life and so impoverish it or disturb the society for a while by a momentary elevation. The truth is that neither the mental effort nor the spiritual impulse can suffice, divorced from each other, to overcome the immense resistance of material Nature. She demands their alliance in a complete effort before she will suffer a complete change in humanity. But, usually, these two great agents are unwilling to make to each other the necessary concessions.

The mental life concentrates on the aesthetic, the ethical and the intellectual activities. Essential mentality is idealistic and a seeker after perfection. The subtle self, the brilliant Atman,[1] is ever a dreamer. A dream of perfect beauty, perfect conduct, perfect Truth, whether seeking new forms of the Eternal or revitalising the old, is the very soul of pure mentality. But it knows not how to deal with the resistance of Matter. There it is hampered and inefficient, works by bungling experiments and has either to withdraw from the struggle or submit to the grey actuality. Or else, by studying the material life and accepting the conditions of the contest, it may succeed, but only in imposing temporarily some artificial system which infinite Nature either rends and casts aside or disfigures out of recognition or by withdrawing her assent leaves as the corpse of a dead ideal. Few and far between have been those realisations of the dreamer in Man which the world has gladly accepted, looks back to with a fond memory and seeks, in its elements, to cherish.

When the gulf between actual life and the temperament of the thinker is too great, we see as the result a sort of withdrawing of the Mind from life in order to act with a greater freedom in its own sphere. The poet living among his brilliant visions, the artist absorbed in his art, the philosopher thinking out the problems of the intellect in his solitary chamber, the scientist, the scholar caring only for their studies and their experiments, were often in former days, are even now not unoften the Sannyasins of the intellect. To the work they have done for humanity, all its past bears record.

But such seclusion is justified only by some special activity. Mind finds fully its force and action only when it casts itself upon life and accepts equally its possibilities and its resistances as the means of a greater self-perfection. In the struggle with the difficulties of the material world the ethical development of the individual is firmly shaped and the great schools of conduct are formed; by contact with the facts of life Art attains to vitality, Thought assures its abstractions, the generalisations of the philosopher base themselves on a stable foundation of science and experience.

This mixing with life may, however, be pursued for the sake of the individual mind and with an entire indifference to the forms of the material existence or the uplifting of the race. This indifference is seen at its highest in the Epicurean discipline and is not entirely absent from the Stoic; and even altruism does the works of compassion more often for its own sake than for the sake of the world it helps. But this too is a limited fulfilment. The progressive mind is seen at its noblest when it strives to elevate the whole race to its own level whether by sowing broadcast the image of its own thought and fulfilment or by changing the material life of the race into fresh forms, religious, intellectual, social or political, intended to represent more nearly that ideal of truth, beauty, justice, righteousness with which the man's own soul is illumined. Failure in such a field matters little; for the mere attempt is dynamic and creative. The struggle of Mind to elevate life is the promise and condition of the conquest of life by that which is higher even than Mind.

That highest thing, the spiritual existence, is concerned with what is eternal but not therefore entirely aloof from the transient. For the spiritual man the mind's dream of perfect beauty is realised in an eternal love, beauty and delight that has no dependence and is equal behind all objective appearances; its dream of perfect Truth in the supreme, self-existent, self-apparent and eternal Verity which never varies, but explains and is the secret of all variations and the goal of all progress; its dream of perfect action in the omnipotent and self-guiding Law that is inherent for ever in all things and translates itself here in the rhythm of the worlds. What is fugitive vision or constant effort of creation in the brilliant Self is an eternally existing Reality in the Self that knows[2] and is the Lord.

But if it is often difficult for the mental life to accommodate itself to the dully resistant material activity, how much more difficult must it seem for the spiritual existence to live on in a world that appears full not of the Truth but of every lie and illusion, not of Love and Beauty but of an encompassing discord and ugliness, not of the Law of Truth but of victorious selfishness and sin? Therefore the spiritual life tends easily in the saint and Sannyasin to withdraw from the material existence and reject it either wholly and physically or in the spirit. It sees this world as the kingdom of evil or of ignorance and the eternal and divine either in a far-off heaven or beyond where there is no world and no life. It separates itself inwardly, if not also physically, from the world's impurities; it asserts the spiritual reality in a spotless isolation. This withdrawal renders an invaluable service to the material life itself by forcing it to regard and even to bow down to something that is the direct negation of its own petty ideals, sordid cares and egoistic self-content.

But the work in the world of so supreme a power as spiritual force cannot be thus limited. The spiritual life also can return upon the material and use it as a means of its own greater fullness. Refusing to be blinded by the dualities, the appearances, it can seek in all appearances whatsoever the vision of the same Lord, the same eternal Truth, Beauty, Love, Delight. The Vedantic formula of the Self in all things, all things in the Self and all things as becomings of the Self is the key to this richer and all-embracing Yoga.

But the spiritual life, like the mental, may thus make use of this outward existence for the benefit of the individual with a perfect indifference to any collective uplifting of the merely symbolic world which it uses. Since the Eternal is for ever the same in all things and all things the same to the Eternal, since the exact mode of action and the result are of no importance compared with the working out in oneself of the one great realisation, this spiritual indifference accepts no matter what environment, no matter what action, dispassionately, prepared to retire as soon as its own supreme end is realised. It is so that many have understood the ideal of the Gita. Or else the inner love and bliss may pour itself out on the world in good deeds, in service, in compassion, the inner Truth in the giving of knowledge, without therefore attempting the transformation of a world which must by its inalienable nature remain a battlefield of the dualities, of sin and virtue, of truth and error, of joy and suffering.

But if Progress also is one of the chief terms of world-existence and a progressive manifestation of the Divine the true sense of Nature, this limitation also is invalid. It is possible for the spiritual life in the world, and it is its real mission, to change the material life into its own image, the image of the Divine. Therefore, besides the great solitaries who have sought and attained their self-liberation, we have the great spiritual teachers who have also liberated others and, supreme of all, the great dynamic souls who, feeling themselves stronger in the might of the Spirit than all the forces of the material life banded together, have thrown themselves upon the world, grappled with it in a loving wrestle and striven to compel its consent to its own transfiguration. Ordinarily, the effort is concentrated on a mental and moral change in humanity, but it may extend itself also to the alteration of the forms of our life and its institutions so that they too may be a better mould for the inpourings of the Spirit. These attempts have been the supreme landmarks in the progressive development of human ideals and the divine preparation of the race. Every one of them, whatever its outward results, has left Earth more capable of Heaven and quickened in its tardy movements the evolutionary Yoga of Nature.

In India, for the last thousand years and more, the spiritual life and the material have existed side by side to the exclusion of the progressive mind. Spirituality has made terms for itself with Matter by renouncing the attempt at general progress. It has obtained from society the right of free spiritual development for all who assume some distinctive symbol, such as the garb of the Sannyasin, the recognition of that life as man's goal and those who live it as worthy of an absolute reverence, and the casting of society itself into such a religious mould that its most customary acts should be accompanied by a formal reminder of the spiritual symbolism of life and its ultimate destination. On the other hand, there was conceded to society the right of inertia and immobile self-conservation. The concession destroyed much of the value of the terms. The religious mould being fixed, the formal reminder tended to become a routine and to lose its living sense. The constant attempts to change the mould by new sects and religions ended only in a new routine or a modification of the old; for the saving element of the free and active mind had been exiled. The material life, handed over to the Ignorance, the purposeless and endless duality, became a leaden and dolorous yoke from which flight was the only escape.

The schools of Indian Yoga lent themselves to the compromise. Individual perfection or liberation was made the aim, seclusion of some kind from the ordinary activities the condition, the renunciation of life the culmination. The teacher gave his knowledge only to a small circle of disciples. Or if a wider movement was attempted, it was still the release of the individual soul that remained the aim. The pact with an immobile society was, for the most part, observed.

The utility of the compromise in the then actual state of the world cannot be doubted. It secured in India a society which lent itself to the preservation and the worship of spirituality, a country apart in which as in a fortress the highest spiritual ideal could maintain itself in its most absolute purity unoverpowered by the siege of the forces around it. But it was a compromise, not an absolute victory. The material life lost the divine impulse to growth, the spiritual preserved by isolation its height and purity, but sacrificed its full power and serviceableness to the world. Therefore, in the divine Providence the country of the Yogins and the Sannyasins has been forced into a strict and imperative contact with the very element it had rejected, the element of the progressive Mind, so that it might recover what was now wanting to it.

We have to recognise once more that the individual exists not in himself alone but in the collectivity and that individual perfection and liberation are not the whole sense of God's intention in the world. The free use of our liberty includes also the liberation of others and of mankind; the perfect utility of our perfection is, having realised in ourselves the divine symbol, to reproduce, multiply and ultimately universalise it in others.

Therefore from a concrete view of human life in its threefold potentialities we come to the same conclusion that we had drawn from an observation of Nature in her general workings and the three steps of her evolution. And we begin to perceive a complete aim for our synthesis of Yoga.

Spirit is the crown of universal existence; Matter is its basis; Mind is the link between the two. Spirit is that which is eternal; Mind and Matter are its workings. Spirit is that which is concealed and has to be revealed; mind and body are the means by which it seeks to reveal itself. Spirit is the image of the Lord of the Yoga; mind and body are the means He has provided for reproducing that image in phenomenal existence. All Nature is an attempt at a progressive revelation of the concealed Truth, a more and more successful reproduction of the divine image.

But what Nature aims at for the mass in a slow evolution, Yoga effects for the individual by a rapid revolution. It works by a quickening of all her energies, a sublimation of all her faculties. While she develops the spiritual life with difficulty and has constantly to fall back from it for the sake of her lower realisations, the sublimated force, the concentrated method of Yoga can attain directly and carry with it the perfection of the mind and even, if she will, the perfection of the body. Nature seeks the Divine in her own symbols: Yoga goes beyond Nature to the Lord of Nature, beyond universe to the Transcendent and can return with the transcendent light and power, with the fiat of the Omnipotent.

But their aim is one in the end. The generalisation of Yoga in humanity must be the last victory of Nature over her own delays and concealments. Even as now by the progressive mind in Science she seeks to make all mankind fit for the full development of the mental life, so by Yoga must she inevitably seek to make all mankind fit for the higher evolution, the second birth, the spiritual existence. And as the mental life uses and perfects the material, so will the spiritual use and perfect the material and the mental existence as the instruments of a divine self-expression. The ages when that is accomplished, are the legendary Satya or Krita[3] Yugas, the ages of the Truth manifested in the symbol, of the great work done when Nature in mankind, illumined, satisfied and blissful, rests in the culmination of her endeavour.

It is for man to know her meaning, no longer misunderstanding, vilifying or misusing the universal Mother, and to aspire always by her mightiest means to her highest ideal.

---

1. Who dwells in Dream, the inly conscious, the enjoyer of abstractions, the Brilliant. Mandukya Upanishad 4.
2. The Unified, in whom conscious thought is concentrated, who is all delight and enjoyer of delight, the Wise. . . . He is the Lord of all, the Omniscient, the inner Guide. Mandukya Upanishad 5, 6.
3. Satya means Truth; Krita, effected or completed.

CHAPTER IV. THE SYSTEMS OF YOGA

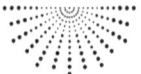

THESE relations between the different psychological divisions of the human being and these various utilities and objects of effort founded on them, such as we have seen them in our brief survey of the natural evolution, we shall find repeated in the fundamental principles and methods of the different schools of Yoga. And if we seek to combine and harmonise their central practices and their predominant aims, we shall find that the basis provided by Nature is still our natural basis and the condition of their synthesis.

In one respect Yoga exceeds the normal operation of cosmic Nature and climbs beyond her. For the aim of the Universal Mother is to embrace the Divine in her own play and creations and there to realise It. But in the highest flights of Yoga she reaches beyond herself and realises the Divine in Itself exceeding the universe and even standing apart from the cosmic play. Therefore by some it is supposed that this is not only the highest but also the one true or exclusively preferable object of Yoga.

Yet it is always through something which she has formed in her evolution that Nature thus overpasses her evolution. It is the individual heart that by sublimating its highest and purest emotions attains to the transcendent Bliss or the ineffable Nirvana, the individual mind that by converting its ordinary functionings into a knowledge beyond mentality knows its oneness with the Ineffable and merges its separate existence in that transcendent unity. And always it is the individual, the Self conditioned in its experience by Nature and working through her formations, that attains to the Self unconditioned, free and transcendent.

In practice three conceptions are necessary before there can be any possibility of Yoga; there must be, as it were, three consenting parties to the effort,—God, Nature and the human soul or, in more abstract language, the Transcendental, the Universal and the Individual. If the individual and Nature are left to themselves, the one is bound to the other and unable to exceed appreciably her lingering march. Something transcendent is needed, free from her and greater, which will act upon us and her, attracting us upward to Itself and securing from her by good grace or by force her consent to the individual ascension.

It is this truth which makes necessary to every philosophy of Yoga the conception of the Ishwara, Lord, supreme Soul or supreme Self, towards whom the effort is directed and who gives the illuminating touch and the strength to attain. Equally true is the complementary idea so often enforced by the Yoga of devotion that as the Transcendent is necessary to the individual and sought after by him, so also the individual is necessary in a sense to the Transcendent and sought after by It. If the Bhakta seeks and yearns after Bhagavan, Bhagavan also seeks and yearns after the Bhakta.[1] There can be no Yoga of knowledge without a human seeker of the knowledge, the supreme subject of knowledge and the divine use by the individual of the universal faculties of knowledge; no Yoga of devotion without the human God-lover, the supreme object of love and delight and the divine use by the individual of the universal faculties of spiritual, emotional and aesthetic enjoyment; no Yoga of works without the human worker, the supreme Will, Master of all works and sacrifices, and the divine use by the individual of the universal faculties of power and action. However Monistic may be our intellectual conception of the highest truth of things, in practice we are compelled to accept this omnipresent Trinity.

For the contact of the human and individual consciousness with the divine is the very essence of Yoga. Yoga is the union of that which has become separated in the play of the universe with its own true self, origin and universality. The contact may take place at any point of the complex and intricately organised consciousness which we call our personality. It may be effected in the physical through the body; in the vital through the action of those functionings which determine the state and the experiences of our nervous being; through the mentality, whether by means of the emotional heart, the active will or the understanding mind, or more largely by a general conversion of the mental consciousness in all its activities. It may equally be accomplished through a direct awakening to the universal or transcendent Truth and Bliss by the conversion of the central ego in the mind. And according to the point of contact that we choose will be the type of the Yoga that we practise.

For if, leaving aside the complexities of their particular processes, we fix our regard on the central principle of the chief schools of Yoga still prevalent in India, we find that they arrange themselves in an ascending order which starts from the lowest rung of the ladder, the body, and ascends to the direct contact between the individual soul and the transcendent and universal Self. Hathayoga selects the body and the vital functionings as its instruments of perfection and realisation; its concern is with the gross body. Rajayoga selects the mental being in its different parts as its lever-power; it concentrates on the subtle body. The triple Path of Works, of Love and of Knowledge uses some part of the mental being, will, heart or intellect as a starting-point and seeks by its conversion to arrive at the liberating Truth, Beatitude and Infinity which are the nature of the spiritual life. Its method is a direct commerce between the human Purusha in the individual body and the divine Purusha who dwells in every body and yet transcends all form and name.

Hathayoga aims at the conquest of the life and the body whose combination in the food sheath and the vital vehicle constitutes, as we have seen, the gross body and whose equilibrium is the foundation of all Nature's workings in the human being. The equilibrium established by Nature is sufficient for the normal egoistic life; it is insufficient for the purpose of the Hathayogin. For it is calculated on the amount of vital or dynamic force necessary to drive the physical engine during the normal span of human life and to perform more or less adequately the various workings demanded of it by the individual life inhabiting this frame and the world-environment by which it is conditioned.

Hathayoga therefore seeks to rectify Nature and establish another equilibrium by which the physical frame will be able to sustain the inrush of an increasing vital or dynamic force of Prana indefinite, almost infinite in its quantity or intensity. In Nature the equilibrium is based upon the individualisation of a limited quantity and force of the Prana; more than that the individual is by personal and hereditary habit unable to bear, use or control. In Hathayoga, the equilibrium opens a door to the universalisation of the individual vitality by admitting into the body, containing, using and controlling a much less fixed and limited action of the universal energy.

The chief processes of Hathayoga are *āsana* and *prāṇāyāma*. By its numerous *āsanas* or fixed postures it first cures the body of that restlessness which is a sign of its inability to contain without working them off in action and movement the vital forces poured into it from the universal Life-Ocean, gives to it an extraordinary health, force and suppleness and seeks to liberate it from the habits by which it is subjected to ordinary physical Nature and kept within the narrow bounds of her normal operations. In the ancient tradition of Hathayoga it has always been supposed that this conquest could be pushed so far even as to conquer to a great extent the force of gravitation. By various subsidiary but elaborate processes the Hathayogin next contrives to keep the body free from all impurities and the nervous system unclogged for those exercises of respiration which are his most important instruments. These are called *prāṇāyāma*, the control of the breath or vital power; for breathing is the chief physical functioning of the vital forces. Pranayama, for the Hathayogin, serves a double purpose. First, it completes the perfection of the body. The vitality is liberated from many of the ordinary necessities of physical Nature; robust health, prolonged youth, often an extraordinary longevity are attained. On the other hand, Pranayama awakens the coiled-up serpent of the Pranic dynamism in the vital sheath and opens to the Yogin fields of consciousness, ranges of experience, abnormal faculties denied to the ordinary human life while it puissantly intensifies such normal powers and faculties as he already possesses.

These advantages can be farther secured and emphasised by other subsidiary processes open to the Hathayogin.

The results of Hathayoga are thus striking to the eye and impose easily on the vulgar or physical mind. And yet at the end we may ask what we have gained at the end of all this stupendous labour. The object of physical Nature, the preservation of the mere physical life, its highest perfection, even in a certain sense the capacity of a greater enjoyment of physical living have been carried out on an abnormal scale. But the weakness of Hathayoga is that its laborious and difficult processes make so great a demand on the time and energy and impose so complete a severance from the ordinary life of men that the utilisation of its results for the life of the world becomes either impracticable or is extraordinarily restricted. If in return for this loss we gain another life in another world within, the mental, the dynamic, these results could have been acquired through other systems, through Rajayoga, through Tantra, by much less laborious methods and held on much less exacting terms. On the other hand the physical results, increased vitality, prolonged youth, health, longevity are of small avail if they must be held by us as misers of ourselves, apart from the common life, for their own sake, not utilised, not thrown into the common sum of the world's activities. Hathayoga attains large results, but at an exorbitant price and to very little purpose.

Rajayoga takes a higher flight. It aims at the liberation and perfection not of the bodily, but of the mental being, the control of the emotional and sensational life, the mastery of the whole apparatus of thought and consciousness. It fixes its eyes on the *citta*, that stuff of mental consciousness in which all these activities arise, and it seeks, even as Hathayoga with its physical material, first to purify and to tranquillise. The normal state of man is a condition of trouble and disorder, a kingdom either at war with itself or badly governed; for the lord, the Purusha, is subjected to his ministers, the faculties, subjected even to his subjects, the instruments of sensation, emotion, action, enjoyment. Swarajya, self-rule, must be substituted for this subjection. First, therefore, the powers of order must be helped to overcome the powers of disorder. The preliminary movement of Rajayoga is a careful self-discipline by which good habits of mind are substituted for the lawless movements that indulge the lower nervous being. By the practice of truth, by renunciation of all forms of egoistic seeking, by abstention from injury to others, by purity, by constant meditation and inclination to the divine Purusha who is the true lord of the mental kingdom, a pure, glad, clear state of mind and heart is established.

This is the first step only. Afterwards, the ordinary activities of the mind and sense must be entirely quieted in order that the soul may be free to ascend to higher states of consciousness and acquire the foundation for a perfect freedom and self-mastery. But Rajayoga does not forget that the disabilities of the ordinary mind proceed largely from its subjection to the reactions of the nervous system and the body. It adopts therefore from the Hathayogic system its devices of *āsana* and *prāṇāyāma*, but reduces their multiple and elaborate forms in each case to one simplest and most directly effective process sufficient for its own immediate object. Thus it gets rid of the Hathayogic complexity and cumbrousness while it utilises the swift and powerful efficacy of its methods for the control of the body and the vital functions and for the awakening of that internal dynamism, full of a latent supernormal faculty, typified in Yogic terminology by the *kuṇḍalinī*, the coiled and sleeping serpent of Energy within. This done, the system proceeds to the perfect quieting of the restless mind and its elevation to a higher plane through concentration of mental force by the successive stages which lead to the utmost inner concentration or ingathered state of the consciousness which is called Samadhi.

By Samadhi, in which the mind acquires the capacity of withdrawing from its limited waking activities into freer and higher states of consciousness, Rajayoga serves a double purpose. It compasses a pure mental action liberated from the confusions of the outer consciousness and passes thence to the higher supra-mental planes on which the individual soul enters into its true spiritual existence. But also it acquires the capacity of that free and concentrated energising of consciousness on its object which our philosophy asserts as the primary cosmic energy and the method of divine action upon the world. By this capacity the Yogin, already possessed of the highest supracosmic knowledge and experience in the state of trance, is able in the waking state to acquire directly whatever knowledge and exercise whatever mastery may be useful or necessary to his activities in the objective world. For the ancient system of Rajayoga aimed not only at Swarajya, self-rule or subjective empire, the entire control by the subjective consciousness of all the states and activities proper to its own domain, but included Samrajya as well, outward empire, the control by the subjective consciousness of its outer activities and environment.

We perceive that as Hathayoga, dealing with the life and body, aims at the supernormal perfection of the physical life and its capacities and goes beyond it into the domain of the mental life, so Rajayoga, operating with the mind, aims at a supernormal perfection and enlargement of the capacities of the mental life and goes beyond it into the domain of the spiritual existence. But the weakness of the system lies in its excessive reliance on abnormal states of trance. This limitation leads first to a certain aloofness from the physical life which is our foundation and the sphere into which we have to bring our mental and spiritual gains. Especially is the spiritual life, in this system, too much associated with the state of Samadhi. Our object is to make the spiritual life and its experiences fully active and fully utilisable in the waking state and even in the normal use of the functions. But in Rajayoga it tends to withdraw into a subliminal plane at the back of our normal experiences instead of descending and possessing our whole existence.

The triple Path of devotion, knowledge and works attempts the province which Rajayoga leaves unoccupied. It differs from Rajayoga in that it does not occupy itself with the elaborate training of the whole mental system as the condition of perfection, but seizes on certain central principles, the intellect, the heart, the will, and seeks to convert their normal operations by turning them away from their ordinary and external preoccupation and activities and concentrating them on the Divine. It differs also in this,—and here from the point of view of an integral Yoga there seems to be a defect,—that it is indifferent to mental and bodily perfection and aims only at purity as a condition of the divine realisation. A second defect is that as actually practised it chooses one of the three parallel paths exclusively and almost in antagonism to the others instead of effecting a synthetic harmony of the intellect, the heart and the will in an integral divine realisation.

The Path of Knowledge aims at the realisation of the unique and supreme Self. It proceeds by the method of intellectual reflection, *vicāra*, to right discrimination, *viveka*. It observes and distinguishes the different elements of our apparent or phenomenal being and rejecting identification with each of them arrives at their exclusion and separation in one common term as constituents of Prakriti, of phenomenal Nature, creations of Maya, the phenomenal consciousness. So it is able to arrive at its right identification with the pure and unique Self which is not mutable or perishable, not determinable by any phenomenon or combination of phenomena. From this point the path, as ordinarily followed, leads to the rejection of the phenomenal worlds from the consciousness as an illusion and the final immergence without return of the individual soul in the Supreme.

But this exclusive consummation is not the sole or inevitable result of the Path of Knowledge. For, followed more largely and with a less individual aim, the method of Knowledge may lead to an active conquest of the cosmic existence for the Divine no less than to a transcendence. The point of this departure is the realisation of the supreme Self not only in one's own being but in all beings and, finally, the realisation of even the phenomenal aspects of the world as a play of the divine consciousness and not something entirely alien to its true nature. And on the basis of this realisation a yet further enlargement is possible, the conversion of all forms of knowledge, however mundane, into activities of the divine consciousness utilisable for the perception of the one and unique Object of knowledge both in itself and through the play of its forms and symbols. Such a method might well lead to the elevation of the whole range of human intellect and perception to the divine level, to its spiritualisation and to the justification of the cosmic travail of knowledge in humanity. The Path of Devotion aims at the enjoyment of the supreme Love and Bliss and utilises normally the conception of the supreme Lord in His personality as the divine Lover and enjoyer of the universe. The world is then realised as a play of the Lord, with our human life as its final stage, pursued through the different phases of self-concealment and self-revelation. The principle of Bhakti Yoga is to utilise all the normal relations of human life into which emotion enters and apply them no longer to transient worldly relations, but to the joy of the All-Loving, the All-Beautiful and the All-Blissful. Worship and meditation are used only for the preparation and increase of intensity of the divine relationship. And this Yoga is catholic in its use of all emotional relations, so that even enmity and opposition to God, considered as an intense, impatient and perverse form of Love, is conceived as a possible means of realisation and salvation. This path, too, as ordinarily practised, leads away from world-existence to an absorption, of another kind than the Monist's, in the Transcendent and Supra-cosmic.

But, here too, the exclusive result is not inevitable. The Yoga itself provides a first corrective by not confining the play of divine love to the relation between the supreme Soul and the individual, but extending it to a common feeling and mutual worship between the devotees themselves united in the same realisation of the supreme Love and Bliss. It provides a yet more general corrective in the realisation of the divine object of Love in all beings not only human but animal, easily extended to all forms whatsoever. We can see how this larger application of the Yoga of Devotion may be so used as to lead to the elevation of the whole range of human emotion, sensation and aesthetic perception to the divine level, its spiritualisation and the justification of the cosmic labour towards love and joy in our humanity.

The Path of Works aims at the dedication of every human activity to the supreme Will. It begins by the renunciation of all egoistic aim for our works, all pursuit of action for an interested aim or for the sake of a worldly result. By this renunciation it so purifies the mind and the will that we become easily conscious of the great universal Energy as the true doer of all our actions and the Lord of that Energy as their ruler and director with the individual as only a mask, an excuse, an instrument or, more positively, a conscious centre of action and phenomenal relation. The choice and direction of the act is more and more consciously left to this supreme Will and this universal Energy. To That our works as well as the results of our works are finally abandoned. The object is the release of the soul from its bondage to appearances and to the reaction of phenomenal activities. Karmayoga is used, like the other paths, to lead to liberation from phenomenal existence and a departure into the Supreme. But here too the exclusive result is not inevitable. The end of the path may be, equally, a perception of the Divine in all energies, in all happenings, in all activities, and a free and unegoistic participation of the soul in the cosmic action. So followed it will lead to the elevation of all human will and activity to the divine level, its spiritualisation and the justification of the cosmic labour towards freedom, power and perfection in the human being.

We can see also that in the integral view of things these three paths are one. Divine Love should normally lead to the perfect knowledge of the Beloved by perfect intimacy, thus becoming a path of Knowledge, and to divine service, thus becoming a path of Works. So also should perfect Knowledge lead to perfect Love and Joy and a full acceptance of the works of That which is known; dedicated Works to the entire love of the Master of the Sacrifice and the deepest knowledge of His ways and His being. It is in this triple path that we come most readily to the absolute knowledge, love and service of the One in all beings and in the entire cosmic manifestation.

---

1. Bhakta, the devotee or lover of God; Bhagavan, God, the Lord of Love and Delight. The third term of the trinity is Bhagavat, the divine revelation of Love.

CHAPTER V. THE SYNTHESIS OF THE SYSTEMS

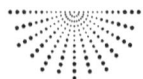

BY THE very nature of the principal Yogic schools, each covering in its operations a part of the complex human integer and attempting to bring out its highest possibilities, it will appear that a synthesis of all of them largely conceived and applied might well result in an integral Yoga. But they are so disparate in their tendencies, so highly specialised and elaborated in their forms, so long confirmed in the mutual opposition of their ideas and methods that we do not easily find how we can arrive at their right union.

An undiscriminating combination in block would not be a synthesis, but a confusion. Nor would a successive practice of each of them in turn be easy in the short span of our human life and with our limited energies, to say nothing of the waste of labour implied in so cumbrous a process. Sometimes, indeed, Hathayoga and Rajayoga are thus successively practised. And in a recent unique example, in the life of Ramakrishna Paramhansa, we see a colossal spiritual capacity first driving straight to the divine realisation, taking, as it were, the kingdom of heaven by violence, and then seizing upon one Yogic method after another and extracting the substance out of it with an incredible rapidity, always to return to the heart of the whole matter, the realisation and possession of God by the power of love, by the extension of inborn spirituality into various experience and by the spontaneous play of an intuitive knowledge. Such an example cannot be generalised. Its object also was special and temporal, to exemplify in the great and decisive experience of a master-soul the truth, now most necessary to humanity, towards which a world long divided into jarring sects and schools is with difficulty labouring, that all sects are forms and fragments of a single integral truth and all disciplines labour in their different ways towards one supreme experience. To know, be and possess the Divine is the one thing needful and it includes or leads up to all the rest; towards this sole good we have to drive and this attained, all the rest that the divine Will chooses for us, all necessary form and manifestation, will be added.

The synthesis we propose cannot, then, be arrived at either by combination in mass or by successive practice. It must therefore be effected by neglecting the forms and outsides of the Yogic disciplines and seizing rather on some central principle common to all which will include and utilise in the right place and proportion their particular principles, and on some central dynamic force which is the common secret of their divergent methods and capable therefore of organising a natural selection and combination of their varied energies and different utilities. This was the aim which we set before ourselves at first when we entered upon our comparative examination of the methods of Nature and the methods of Yoga and we now return to it with the possibility of hazarding some definite solution.

We observe, first, that there still exists in India a remarkable Yogic system which is in its nature synthetical and starts from a great central principle of Nature, a great dynamic force of Nature; but it is a Yoga apart, not a synthesis of other schools. This system is the way of the Tantra. Owing to certain of its developments Tantra has fallen into discredit with those who are not Tantrics; and especially owing to the developments of its left-hand path, the Vama Marga, which not content with exceeding the duality of virtue and sin and instead of replacing them by spontaneous rightness of action seemed, sometimes, to make a method of self-indulgence, a method of unrestrained social immorality. Nevertheless, in its origin, Tantra was a great and puissant system founded upon ideas which were at least partially true. Even its twofold division into the right-hand and left-hand paths, Dakshina Marga and Vama Marga, started from a certain profound perception. In the ancient symbolic sense of the words Dakshina and Vama, it was the distinction between the way of Knowledge and the way of Ananda,—Nature in man liberating itself by right discrimination in power and practice of its own energies, elements and potentialities and Nature in man liberating itself by joyous acceptance in power and practice of its own energies, elements and potentialities. But in both paths there was in the end an obscuration of principles, a deformation of symbols and a fall.

If, however, we leave aside, here also, the actual methods and practices and seek for the central principle, we find, first, that Tantra expressly differentiates itself from the Vedic methods of Yoga. In a sense, all the schools we have hitherto examined are Vedantic in their principle; their force is in knowledge, their method is knowledge, though it is not always discernment by the intellect, but may be, instead, the knowledge of the heart expressed in love and faith or a knowledge in the will working out through action. In all of them the lord of the Yoga is the Purusha, the Conscious Soul that knows, observes, attracts, governs. But in Tantra it is rather Prakriti, the Nature-Soul, the Energy, the Will-in-Power executive in the universe. It was by learning and applying the intimate secrets of this Will-in-Power, its method, its Tantra, that the Tantric Yogin pursued the aims of his discipline,—mastery, perfection, liberation, beatitude. Instead of drawing back from manifested Nature and its difficulties, he confronted them, seized and conquered. But in the end, as is the general tendency of Prakriti, Tantric Yoga largely lost its principle in its machinery and became a thing of formulae and occult mechanism still powerful when rightly used but fallen from the clarity of their original intention.

We have in this central Tantric conception one side of the truth, the worship of the Energy, the Shakti, as the sole effective force for all attainment. We get the other extreme in the Vedantic conception of the Shakti as a power of Illusion and in the search after the silent inactive Purusha as the means of liberation from the deceptions created by the active Energy. But in the integral conception the Conscious Soul is the Lord, the Nature-Soul is his executive Energy. Purusha is of the nature of Sat, the being of conscious self-existence pure and infinite; Shakti or Prakriti is of the nature of Chit,—it is power of the Purusha's self-conscious existence, pure and infinite. The relation of the two exists between the poles of rest and action. When the Energy is absorbed in the bliss of conscious self-existence, there is rest; when the Purusha pours itself out in the action of its Energy, there is action, creation and the enjoyment or Ananda of becoming. But if Ananda is the creator and begetter of all becoming, its method is Tapas or force of the Purusha's consciousness dwelling upon its own infinite potentiality in existence and producing from it truths of conception or real Ideas, *vijñāna*, which, proceeding from an omniscient and omnipotent Self-existence, have the surety of their own fulfilment and contain in themselves the nature and law of their own becoming in the terms of mind, life and matter. The eventual omnipotence of Tapas and the infallible fulfilment of the Idea are the very foundation of all Yoga. In man we render these terms by Will and Faith,—a will that is eventually self-effective because it is of the substance of Knowledge and a faith that is the reflex in the lower consciousness of a Truth or real Idea yet unrealised in the manifestation. It is this self-certainty of the Idea which is meant by the Gita when it says, *yo yac-chraddhaḥ sa eva saḥ*, "whatever is a man's faith or the sure Idea in him, that he becomes."

We see, then, what from the psychological point of view,—and Yoga is nothing but practical psychology,—is the conception of Nature from which we have to start. It is the self-fulfilment of the Purusha through his Energy. But the movement of Nature is twofold, higher and lower, or, as we may choose to term it, divine and undivine. The distinction exists indeed for practical purposes only; for there is nothing that is not divine, and in a larger view it is as meaningless, verbally, as the distinction between natural and supernatural, for all things that are are natural. All things are in Nature and all things are in God. But, for practical purposes, there is a real distinction. The lower Nature, that which we know and are and must remain so long as the faith in us is not changed, acts through limitation and division, is of the nature of Ignorance and culminates in the life of the ego; but the higher Nature, that to which we aspire, acts by unification and transcendence of limitation, is of the nature of Knowledge and culminates in the life divine. The passage from the lower to the higher is the aim of Yoga; and this passage may effect itself by the rejection of the lower and escape into the higher,—the ordinary view-point,—or by the transformation of the lower and its elevation to the higher Nature. It is this, rather, that must be the aim of an integral Yoga.

But in either case it is always through something in the lower that we must rise into the higher existence, and the schools of Yoga each select their own point of departure or their own gate of escape. They specialise certain activities of the lower Prakriti and turn them towards the Divine. But the normal action of Nature in us is an integral movement in which the full complexity of all our elements is affected by and affects all our environments. The whole of life is the Yoga of Nature. The Yoga that we seek must also be an integral action of Nature, and the whole difference between the Yogin and the natural man will be this, that the Yogin seeks to substitute in himself for the integral action of the lower Nature working in and by ego and division the integral action of the higher Nature working in and by God and unity. If indeed our aim be only an escape from the world to God, synthesis is unnecessary and a waste of time; for then our sole practical aim must be to find out one path out of the thousand that lead to God, one shortest possible of short cuts, and not to linger exploring different paths that end in the same goal. But if our aim be a transformation of our integral being into the terms of God-existence, it is then that a synthesis becomes necessary.

The method we have to pursue, then, is to put our whole conscious being into relation and contact with the Divine and to call Him in to transform our entire being into His. Thus in a sense God Himself, the real Person in us, becomes the sadhaka of the sadhana[1] as well as the Master of the Yoga by whom the lower personality is used as the centre of a divine transfiguration and the instrument of its own perfection. In effect, the pressure of the Tapas, the force of consciousness in us dwelling in the Idea of the divine Nature upon that which we are in our entirety, produces its own realisation. The divine and all-knowing and all-effecting descends upon the limited and obscure, progressively illumines and energises the whole lower nature and substitutes its own action for all the terms of the inferior human light and mortal activity.

In psychological fact this method translates itself into the progressive surrender of the ego with its whole field and all its apparatus to the Beyond-ego with its vast and incalculable but always inevitable workings. Certainly, this is no short cut or easy sadhana. It requires a colossal faith, an absolute courage and above all an unflinching patience. For it implies three stages of which only the last can be wholly blissful or rapid,—the attempt of the ego to enter into contact with the Divine, the wide, full and therefore laborious preparation of the whole lower Nature by the divine working to receive and become the higher Nature, and the eventual transformation. In fact, however, the divine Strength, often unobserved and behind the veil, substitutes itself for our weakness and supports us through all our failings of faith, courage and patience. It "makes the blind to see and the lame to stride over the hills." The intellect becomes aware of a Law that beneficently insists and a succour that upholds; the heart speaks of a Master of all things and Friend of man or a universal Mother who upholds through all stumblings. Therefore this path is at once the most difficult imaginable and yet, in comparison with the magnitude of its effort and object, the most easy and sure of all.

There are three outstanding features of this action of the higher when it works integrally on the lower nature. In the first place it does not act according to a fixed system and succession as in the specialised methods of Yoga, but with a sort of free, scattered and yet gradually intensive and purposeful working determined by the temperament of the individual in whom it operates, the helpful materials which his nature offers and the obstacles which it presents to purification and perfection. In a sense, therefore, each man in this path has his own method of Yoga. Yet are there certain broad lines of working common to all which enable us to construct not indeed a routine system, but yet some kind of Shastra or scientific method of the synthetic Yoga.

Secondly, the process, being integral, accepts our nature such as it stands organised by our past evolution and without rejecting anything essential compels all to undergo a divine change. Everything in us is seized by the hands of a mighty Artificer and transformed into a clear image of that which it now seeks confusedly to present. In that ever-progressive experience we begin to perceive how this lower manifestation is constituted and that everything in it, however seemingly deformed or petty or vile, is the more or less distorted or imperfect figure of some element or action in the harmony of the divine Nature. We begin to understand what the Vedic Rishis meant when they spoke of the human forefathers fashioning the gods as a smith forges the crude material in his smithy.

Thirdly, the divine Power in us uses all life as the means of this integral Yoga. Every experience and outer contact with our world-environment, however trifling or however disastrous, is used for the work, and every inner experience, even to the most repellent suffering or the most humiliating fall, becomes a step on the path to perfection. And we recognise in ourselves with opened eyes the method of God in the world, His purpose of light in the obscure, of might in the weak and fallen, of delight in what is grievous and miserable. We see the divine method to be the same in the lower and in the higher working; only in the one it is pursued tardily and obscurely through the subconscious in Nature, in the other it becomes swift and self-conscious and the instrument confesses the hand of the Master. All life is a Yoga of Nature seeking to manifest God within itself. Yoga marks the stage at which this effort becomes capable of self-awareness and therefore of right completion in the individual. It is a gathering up and concentration of the movements dispersed and loosely combined in the lower evolution.

An integral method and an integral result. First, an integral realisation of Divine Being; not only a realisation of the One in its indistinguishable unity, but also in its multitude of aspects which are also necessary to the complete knowledge of it by the relative consciousness; not only realisation of unity in the Self, but of unity in the infinite diversity of activities, worlds and creatures.

Therefore, also, an integral liberation. Not only the freedom born of unbroken contact and identification of the individual being in all its parts with the Divine, *sāyujya-mukti*, by which it can become free[2] even in its separation, even in the duality; not only the *sālokya-mukti* by which the whole conscious existence dwells in the same status of being as the Divine, in the state of Sachchidananda; but also the acquisition of the divine nature by the transformation of this lower being into the human image of the Divine, *sādharmya-mukti*, and the complete and final release of all, the liberation of the consciousness from the transitory mould of the ego and its unification with the One Being, universal both in the world and the individual and transcendentally one both in the world and beyond all universe.

By this integral realisation and liberation, the perfect harmony of the results of Knowledge, Love and Works. For there is attained the complete release from ego and identification in being with the One in all and beyond all. But since the attaining consciousness is not limited by its attainment, we win also the unity in Beatitude and the harmonised diversity in Love, so that all relations of the play remain possible to us even while we retain on the heights of our being the eternal oneness with the Beloved. And by a similar wideness, being capable of a freedom in spirit that embraces life and does not depend upon withdrawal from life, we are able to become without egoism, bondage or reaction the channel in our mind and body for a divine action poured out freely upon the world.

The divine existence is of the nature not only of freedom, but of purity, beatitude and perfection. An integral purity which shall enable on the one hand the perfect reflection of the divine Being in ourselves and on the other the perfect outpouring of its Truth and Law in us in the terms of life and through the right functioning of the complex instrument we are in our outer parts, is the condition of an integral liberty. Its result is an integral beatitude, in which there becomes possible at once the Ananda of all that is in the world seen as symbols of the Divine and the Ananda of that which is not-world. And it prepares the integral perfection of our humanity as a type of the Divine in the conditions of the human manifestation, a perfection founded on a certain free universality of being, of love and joy, of play of knowledge and of play of will in power and will in unegoistic action. This integrality also can be attained by the integral Yoga.

Perfection includes perfection of mind and body, so that the highest results of Rajayoga and Hathayoga should be contained in the widest formula of the synthesis finally to be effected by mankind. At any rate a full development of the general mental and physical faculties and experiences attainable by humanity through Yoga must be included in the scope of the integral method. Nor would these have any *raison d'être* unless employed for an integral mental and physical life. Such a mental and physical life would be in its nature a translation of the spiritual existence into its right mental and physical values. Thus we would arrive at a synthesis of the three degrees of Nature and of the three modes of human existence which she has evolved or is evolving. We would include in the scope of our liberated being and perfected modes of activity the material life, our base, and the mental life, our intermediate instrument.

Nor would the integrality to which we aspire be real or even possible, if it were confined to the individual. Since our divine perfection embraces the realisation of ourselves in being, in life and in love through others as well as through ourselves, the extension of our liberty and of its results in others would be the inevitable outcome as well as the broadest utility of our liberation and perfection. And the constant and inherent attempt of such an extension would be towards its increasing and ultimately complete generalisation in mankind.

The divinising of the normal material life of man and of his great secular attempt of mental and moral self-culture in the individual and the race by this integralisation of a widely perfect spiritual existence would thus be the crown alike of our individual and of our common effort. Such a consummation being no other than the kingdom of heaven within reproduced in the kingdom of heaven without, would be also the true fulfilment of the great dream cherished in different terms by the world's religions.

The widest synthesis of perfection possible to thought is the sole effort entirely worthy of those whose dedicated vision perceives that God dwells concealed in humanity.

---

1. *Sādhana*, the practice by which perfection, *siddhi*, is attained; *sādhaka*, the Yogin who seeks by that practice the *siddhi*.
2. As the Jivanmukta, who is entirely free even without dissolution of the bodily life in a final Samadhi.

THE YOGA OF DIVINE WORKS

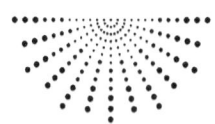

CHAPTER I. THE FOUR AIDS

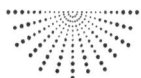

YOGA-SIDDHI, the perfection that comes from the practice of Yoga, can be best attained by the combined working of four great instruments. There is, first, the knowledge of the truths, principles, powers and processes that govern the realisation—*śāstra*. Next comes a patient and persistent action on the lines laid down by this knowledge, the force of our personal effort—*utsāha*. There intervenes, third, uplifting our knowledge and effort into the domain of spiritual experience, the direct suggestion, example and influence of the Teacher—*guru*. Last comes the instrumentality of Time—*kāla*; for in all things there is a cycle of their action and a period of the divine movement.

The supreme Shastra of the integral Yoga is the eternal Veda secret in the heart of every thinking and living being. The lotus of the eternal knowledge and the eternal perfection is a bud closed and folded up within us. It opens swiftly or gradually, petal by petal, through successive realisations, once the mind of man begins to turn towards the Eternal, once his heart, no longer compressed and confined by attachment to finite appearances, becomes enamoured, in whatever degree, of the Infinite. All life, all thought, all energising of the faculties, all experiences passive or active, become thenceforward so many shocks which disintegrate the teguments of the soul and remove the obstacles to the inevitable efflorescence. He who chooses the Infinite has been chosen by the Infinite. He has received the divine touch without which there is no awakening, no opening of the spirit; but once it is received, attainment is sure, whether conquered swiftly in the course of one human life or pursued patiently through many stadia of the cycle of existence in the manifested universe. Nothing can be taught to the mind which is not already concealed as potential knowledge in the unfolding soul of the creature. So also all perfection of which the outer man is capable, is only a realising of the eternal perfection of the Spirit within him. We know the Divine and become the Divine, because we are That already in our secret nature. All teaching is a revealing, all becoming is an unfolding. Self-attainment is the secret; self-knowledge and an increasing consciousness are the means and the process.

The usual agency of this revealing is the Word, the thing heard (*śruta*). The Word may come to us from within; it may come to us from without. But in either case, it is only an agency for setting the hidden knowledge to work. The word within may be the utterance of the inmost soul in us which is always open to the Divine; or it may be the word of the secret and universal Teacher who is seated in the hearts of all. There are rare cases in which none other is needed, for all the rest of the Yoga is an unfolding under that constant touch and guidance; the lotus of the knowledge discloses itself from within by the power of irradiating effulgence which proceeds from the Dweller in the lotus of the heart. Great indeed, but few are those to whom self-knowledge from within is thus sufficient and who do not need to pass under the dominant influence of a written book or a living teacher.

Ordinarily, the Word from without, representative of the Divine, is needed as an aid in the work of self-unfolding; and it may be either a word from the past or the more powerful word of the living Guru. In some cases this representative word is only taken as a sort of excuse for the inner power to awaken and manifest; it is, as it were, a concession of the omnipotent and omniscient Divine to the generality of a law that governs Nature. Thus it is said in the Upanishads of Krishna, son of Devaki, that he received a word of the Rishi Ghora and had the knowledge. So Ramakrishna, having attained by his own internal effort the central illumination, accepted several teachers in the different paths of Yoga, but always showed in the manner and swiftness of his realisation that this acceptance was a concession to the general rule by which effective knowledge must be received as by a disciple from a Guru.

But usually the representative influence occupies a much larger place in the life of the sadhaka. If the Yoga is guided by a received written Shastra,—some Word from the past which embodies the experience of former Yogins,—it may be practised either by personal effort alone or with the aid of a Guru. The spiritual knowledge is then gained through meditation on the truths that are taught and it is made living and conscious by their realisation in the personal experience; the Yoga proceeds by the results of prescribed methods taught in a Scripture or a tradition and reinforced and illumined by the instructions of the Master. This is a narrower practice, but safe and effective within its limits, because it follows a well-beaten track to a long familiar goal.

For the sadhaka of the integral Yoga it is necessary to remember that no written Shastra, however great its authority or however large its spirit, can be more than a partial expression of the eternal Knowledge. He will use, but never bind himself even by the greatest Scripture. Where the Scripture is profound, wide, catholic, it may exercise upon him an influence for the highest good and of incalculable importance. It may be associated in his experience with his awakening to crowning verities and his realisation of the highest experiences. His Yoga may be governed for a long time by one Scripture or by several successively,—if it is in the line of the great Hindu tradition, by the Gita, for example, the Upanishads, the Veda. Or it may be a good part of his development to include in its material a richly varied experience of the truths of many Scriptures and make the future opulent with all that is best in the past. But in the end he must take his station, or better still, if he can, always and from the beginning he must live in his own soul beyond the limitations of the word that he uses. The Gita itself thus declares that the Yogin in his progress must pass beyond the written Truth,—*śabdabrahmātivartate*—beyond all that he has heard and all that he has yet to hear,—*śrotavyasya śrutasya ca*. For he is not the sadhaka of a book or of many books; he is a sadhaka of the Infinite.

Another kind of Shastra is not Scripture, but a statement of the science and methods, the effective principles and way of working of the path of Yoga which the sadhaka elects to follow. Each path has its Shastra, either written or traditional, passing from mouth to mouth through a long line of Teachers. In India a great authority, a high reverence even is ordinarily attached to the written or traditional teaching. All the lines of the Yoga are supposed to be fixed and the Teacher who has received the Shastra by tradition and realised it in practice guides the disciple along the immemorial tracks. One often even hears the objection urged against a new practice, a new Yogic teaching, the adoption of a new formula, "It is not according to the Shastra." But neither in fact nor in the actual practice of the Yogins is there really any such entire rigidity of an iron door shut against new truth, fresh revelation, widened experience. The written or traditional teaching expresses the knowledge and experiences of many centuries systematised, organised, made attainable to the beginner. Its importance and utility are therefore immense. But a great freedom of variation and development is always practicable. Even so highly scientific a system as Rajayoga can be practised on other lines than the organised method of Patanjali. Each of the three paths of the *trimārga*[1] breaks into many bypaths which meet again at the goal. The general knowledge on which the Yoga depends is fixed, but the order, the succession, the devices, the forms must be allowed to vary; for the needs and particular impulsions of the individual nature have to be satisfied even while the general truths remain firm and constant.

An integral and synthetic Yoga needs especially not to be bound by any written or traditional Shastra; for while it embraces the knowledge received from the past, it seeks to organise it anew for the present and the future. An absolute liberty of experience and of the restatement of knowledge in new terms and new combinations is the condition of its self-formation.

Seeking to embrace all life in itself, it is in the position not of a pilgrim following the highroad to his destination, but, to that extent at least, of a path-finder hewing his way through a virgin forest. For Yoga has long diverged from life and the ancient systems which sought to embrace it, such as those of our Vedic forefathers, are far away from us, expressed in terms which are no longer accessible, thrown into forms which are no longer applicable. Since then mankind has moved forward on the current of eternal Time and the same problem has to be approached from a new starting-point.

By this Yoga we not only seek the Infinite, but we call upon the Infinite to unfold himself in human life. Therefore the Shastra of our Yoga must provide for an infinite liberty in the receptive human soul. A free adaptability in the manner and the type of the individual's acceptance of the Universal and Transcendent into himself is the right condition for the full spiritual life in man. Vivekananda, pointing out that the unity of all religions must necessarily express itself by an increasing richness of variety in its forms, said once that the perfect state of that essential unity would come when each man had his own religion, when not bound by sect or traditional form he followed the free self-adaptation of his nature in its relations with the Supreme. So also one may say that the perfection of the integral Yoga will come when each man is able to follow his own path of Yoga, pursuing the development of his own nature in its upsurging towards that which transcends the nature. For freedom is the final law and the last consummation.

Meanwhile certain general lines have to be formed which may help to guide the thought and practice of the sadhaka. But these must take as much as possible the form of general truths, general statements of principle, the most powerful broad directions of effort and development rather than a fixed system which has to be followed as a routine. All Shastra is the outcome of past experience and a help to future experience. It is an aid and a partial guide. It puts up signposts, gives the names of the main roads and the already explored directions, so that the traveller may know whither and by what paths he is proceeding.

The rest depends on personal effort and experience and upon the power of the Guide.

The development of the experience in its rapidity, its amplitude, the intensity and power of its results, depends primarily, in the beginning of the path and long after, on the aspiration and personal effort of the sadhaka. The process of Yoga is a turning of the human soul from the egoistic state of consciousness absorbed in the outward appearances and attractions of things to a higher state in which the Transcendent and Universal can pour itself into the individual mould and transform it. The first determining element of the siddhi is, therefore, the intensity of the turning, the force which directs the soul inward. The power of aspiration of the heart, the force of the will, the concentration of the mind, the perseverance and determination of the applied energy are the measure of that intensity. The ideal sadhaka should be able to say in the Biblical phrase, "My zeal for the Lord has eaten me up." It is this zeal for the Lord,—*utsāha*, the zeal of the whole nature for its divine results, *vyākulatā*, the heart's eagerness for the attainment of the Divine,—that devours the ego and breaks up the limitations of its petty and narrow mould for the full and wide reception of that which it seeks, that which, being universal, exceeds and, being transcendent, surpasses even the largest and highest individual self and nature.

But this is only one side of the force that works for perfection. The process of the integral Yoga has three stages, not indeed sharply distinguished or separate, but in a certain measure successive. There must be, first, the effort towards at least an initial and enabling self-transcendence and contact with the Divine; next, the reception of that which transcends, that with which we have gained communion, into ourselves for the transformation of our whole conscious being; last, the utilisation of our transformed humanity as a divine centre in the world. So long as the contact with the Divine is not in some considerable degree established, so long as there is not some measure of sustained identity, *sāyujya*, the element of personal effort must normally predominate. But in proportion as this contact establishes itself, the sadhaka must become conscious that a force other than his own, a force transcending his egoistic endeavour and capacity, is at work in him and to this Power he learns progressively to submit himself and delivers up to it the charge of his Yoga. In the end his own will and force become one with the higher Power; he merges them in the divine Will and its transcendent and universal Force. He finds it thenceforward presiding over the necessary transformation of his mental, vital and physical being with an impartial wisdom and provident effectivity of which the eager and interested ego is not capable. It is when this identification and this self-merging are complete that the divine centre in the world is ready. Purified, liberated, plastic, illumined, it can begin to serve as a means for the direct action of a supreme Power in the larger Yoga of humanity or superhumanity, of the earth's spiritual progression or its transformation.

Always indeed it is the higher Power that acts. Our sense of personal effort and aspiration comes from the attempt of the egoistic mind to identify itself in a wrong and imperfect way with the workings of the divine Force. It persists in applying to experience on a supernormal plane the ordinary terms of mentality which it applies to its normal experiences in the world. In the world we act with the sense of egoism; we claim the universal forces that work in us as our own; we claim as the effect of our personal will, wisdom, force, virtue the selective, formative, progressive action of the Transcendent in this frame of mind, life and body. Enlightenment brings to us the knowledge that the ego is only an instrument; we begin to perceive and feel that these things are our own in the sense that they belong to our supreme and integral Self, one with the Transcendent, not to the instrumental ego. Our limitations and distortions are our contribution to the working; the true power in it is the Divine's. When the human ego realises that its will is a tool, its wisdom ignorance and childishness, its power an infant's groping, its virtue a pretentious impurity, and learns to trust itself to that which transcends it, that is its salvation. The apparent freedom and self-assertion of our personal being to which we are so profoundly attached, conceal a most pitiable subjection to a thousand suggestions, impulsions, forces which we have made extraneous to our little person. Our ego, boasting of freedom, is at every moment the slave, toy and puppet of countless beings, powers, forces, influences in universal Nature. The self-abnegation of the ego in the Divine is its self-fulfilment; its surrender to that which transcends it is its liberation from bonds and limits and its perfect freedom.

But still, in the practical development, each of the three stages has its necessity and utility and must be given its time or its place. It will not do, it cannot be safe or effective to begin with the last and highest alone. It would not be the right course, either, to leap prematurely from one to another. For even if from the beginning we recognise in mind and heart the Supreme, there are elements of the nature which long prevent the recognition from becoming realisation. But without realisation our mental belief cannot become a dynamic reality; it is still only a figure of knowledge, not a living truth, an idea, not yet a power. And even if realisation has begun, it may be dangerous to imagine or to assume too soon that we are altogether in the hands of the Supreme or are acting as his instrument. That assumption may introduce a calamitous falsity; it may produce a helpless inertia or, magnifying the movements of the ego with the Divine Name, it may disastrously distort and ruin the whole course of the Yoga. There is a period, more or less prolonged, of internal effort and struggle in which the individual will has to reject the darkness and distortions of the lower nature and to put itself resolutely or vehemently on the side of the divine Light. The mental energies, the heart's emotions, the vital desires, the very physical being have to be compelled into the right attitude or trained to admit and answer to the right influences. It is only then, only when this has been truly done, that the surrender of the lower to the higher can be effected, because the sacrifice has become acceptable.

The personal will of the sadhaka has first to seize on the egoistic energies and turn them towards the light and the right; once turned, he has still to train them to recognise that always, always to accept, always to follow that. Progressing, he learns, still using the personal will, personal effort, personal energies, to employ them as representatives of the higher Power and in conscious obedience to the higher Influence. Progressing yet farther, his will, effort, energy become no longer personal and separate, but activities of that higher Power and Influence at work in the individual. But there is still a sort of gulf or distance which necessitates an obscure process of transit, not always accurate, sometimes even very distorting, between the divine Origin and the emerging human current. At the end of the process, with the progressive disappearance of egoism and impurity and ignorance, this last separation is removed; all in the individual becomes the divine working.

As the supreme Shastra of the integral Yoga is the eternal Veda secret in the heart of every man, so its supreme Guide and Teacher is the inner Guide, the World-Teacher, *jagad-guru*, secret within us. It is he who destroys our darkness by the resplendent light of his knowledge; that light becomes within us the increasing glory of his own self-revelation. He discloses progressively in us his own nature of freedom, bliss, love, power, immortal being. He sets above us his divine example as our ideal and transforms the lower existence into a reflection of that which it contemplates. By the inpouring of his own influence and presence into us he enables the individual being to attain to identity with the universal and transcendent.

What is his method and his system? He has no method and every method. His system is a natural organisation of the highest processes and movements of which the nature is capable. Applying themselves even to the pettiest details and to the actions the most insignificant in their appearance with as much care and thoroughness as to the greatest, they in the end lift all into the Light and transform all. For in his Yoga there is nothing too small to be used and nothing too great to be attempted. As the servant and disciple of the Master has no business with pride or egoism because all is done for him from above, so also he has no right to despond because of his personal deficiencies or the stumblings of his nature. For the Force that works in him is impersonal—or superpersonal—and infinite.

The full recognition of this inner Guide, Master of the Yoga, lord, light, enjoyer and goal of all sacrifice and effort, is of the utmost importance in the path of integral perfection. It is immaterial whether he is first seen as an impersonal Wisdom, Love and Power behind all things, as an Absolute manifesting in the relative and attracting it, as one's highest Self and the highest Self of all, as a Divine Person within us and in the world, in one of his—or her—numerous forms and names or as the ideal which the mind conceives. In the end we perceive that he is all and more than all these things together. The mind's door of entry to the conception of him must necessarily vary according to the past evolution and the present nature.

This inner Guide is often veiled at first by the very intensity of our personal effort and by the ego's preoccupation with itself and its aims. As we gain in clarity and the turmoil of egoistic effort gives place to a calmer self-knowledge, we recognise the source of the growing light within us. We recognise it retrospectively as we realise how all our obscure and conflicting movements have been determined towards an end that we only now begin to perceive, how even before our entrance into the path of the Yoga the evolution of our life has been designedly led towards its turning-point. For now we begin to understand the sense of our struggles and efforts, successes and failures. At last we are able to seize the meaning of our ordeals and sufferings and can appreciate the help that was given us by all that hurt and resisted and the utility of our very falls and stumblings. We recognise this divine leading afterwards, not retrospectively but immediately, in the moulding of our thoughts by a transcendent Seer, of our will and actions by an all-embracing Power, of our emotional life by an all-attracting and all-assimilating Bliss and Love. We recognise it too in a more personal relation that from the first touched or at the last seizes us; we feel the eternal presence of a supreme Master, Friend, Lover, Teacher. We recognise it in the essence of our being as that develops into likeness and oneness with a greater and wider existence; for we perceive that this miraculous development is not the result of our own efforts: an eternal Perfection is moulding us into its own image. One who is the Lord or Ishwara of the Yogic philosophies, the Guide in the conscious being (*caitya guru* or *antaryāmin*), the Absolute of the thinker, the Unknowable of the Agnostic, the universal Force of the materialist, the supreme Soul and the supreme Shakti, the One who is differently named and imaged by the religions, is the Master of our Yoga.

To see, know, become and fulfil this One in our inner selves and in all our outer nature, was always the secret goal and becomes now the conscious purpose of our embodied existence. To be conscious of him in all parts of our being and equally in all that the dividing mind sees as outside our being, is the consummation of the individual consciousness. To be possessed by him and possess him in ourselves and in all things is the term of all empire and mastery. To enjoy him in all experience of passivity and activity, of peace and of power, of unity and of difference is the happiness which the Jiva, the individual soul manifested in the world, is obscurely seeking. This is the entire definition of the aim of integral Yoga; it is the rendering in personal experience of the truth which universal Nature has hidden in herself and which she travails to discover. It is the conversion of the human soul into the divine soul and of natural life into divine living.

~

The surest way towards this integral fulfilment is to find the Master of the secret who dwells within us, open ourselves constantly to the divine Power which is also the divine Wisdom and Love and trust to it to effect the conversion. But it is difficult for the egoistic consciousness to do this at all at the beginning. And, if done at all, it is still difficult to do it perfectly and in every strand of our nature. It is difficult at first because our egoistic habits of thought, of sensation, of feeling block up the avenues by which we can arrive at the perception that is needed. It is difficult afterwards because the faith, the surrender, the courage requisite in this path are not easy to the ego-clouded soul. The divine working is not the working which the egoistic mind desires or approves; for it uses error in order to arrive at truth, suffering in order to arrive at bliss, imperfection in order to arrive at perfection. The ego cannot see where it is being led; it revolts against the leading, loses confidence, loses courage. These failings would not matter; for the divine Guide within is not offended by our revolt, not discouraged by our want of faith or repelled by our weakness; he has the entire love of the mother and the entire patience of the teacher. But by withdrawing our assent from the guidance we lose the consciousness, though not all the actuality—not, in any case, the eventuality—of its benefit. And we withdraw our assent because we fail to distinguish our higher Self from the lower through which he is preparing his self-revelation. As in the world, so in ourselves, we cannot see God because of his workings and, especially, because he works in us through our nature and not by a succession of arbitrary miracles. Man demands miracles that he may have faith; he wishes to be dazzled in order that he may see. And this impatience, this ignorance may turn into a great danger and disaster if, in our revolt against the divine leading, we call in another distorting Force more satisfying to our impulses and desires and ask it to guide us and give it the Divine Name.

But while it is difficult for man to believe in something unseen within himself, it is easy for him to believe in something which he can image as extraneous to himself. The spiritual progress of most human beings demands an extraneous support, an object of faith outside us. It needs an external image of God; or it needs a human representative,—Incarnation, Prophet or Guru; or it demands both and receives them. For according to the need of the human soul the Divine manifests himself as deity, as human divine or in simple humanity—using that thick disguise, which so successfully conceals the Godhead, for a means of transmission of his guidance.

The Hindu discipline of spirituality provides for this need of the soul by the conceptions of the Ishta Devata, the Avatar and the Guru. By the Ishta Devata, the chosen deity, is meant,—not some inferior Power, but a name and form of the transcendent and universal Godhead. Almost all religions either have as their base or make use of some such name and form of the Divine. Its necessity for the human soul is evident. God is the All and more than the All. But that which is more than the All, how shall man conceive? And even the All is at first too hard for him; for he himself in his active consciousness is a limited and selective formation and can open himself only to that which is in harmony with his limited nature. There are things in the All which are too hard for his comprehension or seem too terrible to his sensitive emotions and cowering sensations. Or, simply, he cannot conceive as the Divine, cannot approach or cannot recognise something that is too much out of the circle of his ignorant or partial conceptions. It is necessary for him to conceive God in his own image or in some form that is beyond himself but consonant with his highest tendencies and seizable by his feelings or his intelligence. Otherwise it would be difficult for him to come into contact and communion with the Divine.

Even then his nature calls for a human intermediary so that he may feel the Divine in something entirely close to his own humanity and sensible in a human influence and example. This call is satisfied by the Divine manifest in a human appearance, the Incarnation, the Avatar—Krishna, Christ, Buddha. Or if this is too hard for him to conceive, the Divine represents himself through a less marvellous intermediary,—Prophet or Teacher. For many who cannot conceive or are unwilling to accept the Divine Man, are ready to open themselves to the supreme man, terming him not incarnation but world-teacher or divine representative.

This also is not enough; a living influence, a living example, a present instruction is needed. For it is only the few who can make the past Teacher and his teaching, the past Incarnation and his example and influence a living force in their lives. For this need also the Hindu discipline provides in the relation of the Guru and the disciple. The Guru may sometimes be the Incarnation or World-Teacher; but it is sufficient that he should represent to the disciple the divine wisdom, convey to him something of the divine ideal or make him feel the realised relation of the human soul with the Eternal.

The sadhaka of the integral Yoga will make use of all these aids according to his nature; but it is necessary that he should shun their limitations and cast from himself that exclusive tendency of egoistic mind which cries, "My God, my Incarnation, my Prophet, my Guru," and opposes it to all other realisation in a sectarian or a fanatical spirit. All sectarianism, all fanaticism must be shunned; for it is inconsistent with the integrity of the divine realisation.

On the contrary, the sadhaka of the integral Yoga will not be satisfied until he has included all other names and forms of Deity in his own conception, seen his own Ishta Devata in all others, unified all Avatars in the unity of Him who descends in the Avatar, welded the truth in all teachings into the harmony of the Eternal Wisdom.

Nor should he forget the aim of these external aids which is to awaken his soul to the Divine within him. Nothing has been finally accomplished if that has not been accomplished. It is not sufficient to worship Krishna, Christ or Buddha without, if there is not the revealing and the formation of the Buddha, the Christ or Krishna in ourselves. And all other aids equally have no other purpose; each is a bridge between man's unconverted state and the revelation of the Divine within him.

The Teacher of the integral Yoga will follow as far as he may the method of the Teacher within us. He will lead the disciple through the nature of the disciple. Teaching, example, influence,—these are the three instruments of the Guru. But the wise Teacher will not seek to impose himself or his opinions on the passive acceptance of the receptive mind; he will throw in only what is productive and sure as a seed which will grow under the divine fostering within. He will seek to awaken much more than to instruct; he will aim at the growth of the faculties and the experiences by a natural process and free expansion. He will give a method as an aid, as a utilisable device, not as an imperative formula or a fixed routine. And he will be on his guard against any turning of the means into a limitation, against the mechanising of process. His whole business is to awaken the divine light and set working the divine force of which he himself is only a means and an aid, a body or a channel.

The example is more powerful than the instruction; but it is not the example of the outward acts nor that of the personal character which is of most importance. These have their place and their utility; but what will most stimulate aspiration in others is the central fact of the divine realisation within him governing his whole life and inner state and all his activities. This is the universal and essential element; the rest belongs to individual person and circumstance. It is this dynamic realisation that the sadhaka must feel and reproduce in himself according to his own nature; he need not strive after an imitation from outside which may well be sterilising rather than productive of right and natural fruits.

Influence is more important than example. Influence is not the outward authority of the Teacher over his disciple, but the power of his contact, of his presence, of the nearness of his soul to the soul of another, infusing into it, even though in silence, that which he himself is and possesses. This is the supreme sign of the Master. For the greatest Master is much less a Teacher than a Presence pouring the divine consciousness and its constituting light and power and purity and bliss into all who are receptive around him.

And it shall also be a sign of the teacher of the integral Yoga that he does not arrogate to himself Guru-hood in a humanly vain and self-exalting spirit. His work, if he has one, is a trust from above, he himself a channel, a vessel or a representative. He is a man helping his brothers, a child leading children, a Light kindling other lights, an awakened Soul awakening souls, at highest a Power or Presence of the Divine calling to him other powers of the Divine.

~

The sadhaka who has all these aids is sure of his goal. Even a fall will be for him only a means of rising and death a passage towards fulfilment. For once on this path, birth and death become only processes in the development of his being and the stages of his journey.

Time is the remaining aid needed for the effectivity of the process. Time presents itself to human effort as an enemy or a friend, as a resistance, a medium or an instrument. But always it is really the instrument of the soul.

Time is a field of circumstances and forces meeting and working out a resultant progression whose course it measures. To the ego it is a tyrant or a resistance, to the Divine an instrument. Therefore, while our effort is personal, Time appears as a resistance, for it presents to us all the obstruction of the forces that conflict with our own. When the divine working and the personal are combined in our consciousness, it appears as a medium and a condition. When the two become one, it appears as a servant and instrument.

The ideal attitude of the sadhaka towards Time is to have an endless patience as if he had all eternity for his fulfilment and yet to develop the energy that shall realise now and with an ever-increasing mastery and pressure of rapidity till it reaches the miraculous instantaneousness of the supreme divine Transformation.

---

1. The triple path of Knowledge, Devotion and Works.

CHAPTER II. SELF-CONSECRATION

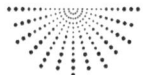

ALL YOGA is in its nature a new birth; it is a birth out of the ordinary, the mentalised material life of man into a higher spiritual consciousness and a greater and diviner being. No Yoga can be successfully undertaken and followed unless there is a strong awakening to the necessity of that larger spiritual existence. The soul that is called to this deep and vast inward change, may arrive in different ways to the initial departure. It may come to it by its own natural development which has been leading it unconsciously towards the awakening; it may reach it through the influence of a religion or the attraction of a philosophy; it may approach it by a slow illumination or leap to it by a sudden touch or shock; it may be pushed or led to it by the pressure of outward circumstances or by an inward necessity, by a single word that breaks the seals of the mind or by long reflection, by the distant example of one who has trod the path or by contact and daily influence. According to the nature and the circumstances the call will come.

But in whatever way it comes, there must be a decision of the mind and the will and, as its result, a complete and effective self-consecration. The acceptance of a new spiritual idea-force and upward orientation in the being, an illumination, a turning or conversion seized on by the will and the heart's aspiration,—this is the momentous act which contains as in a seed all the results that the Yoga has to give. The mere idea or intellectual seeking of something higher beyond, however strongly grasped by the mind's interest, is ineffective unless it is seized on by the heart as the one thing desirable and by the will as the one thing to be done. For truth of the Spirit has not to be merely thought but to be lived, and to live it demands a unified single-mindedness of the being; so great a change as is contemplated by the Yoga is not to be effected by a divided will or by a small portion of the energy or by a hesitating mind. He who seeks the Divine must consecrate himself to God and to God only.

If the change comes suddenly and decisively by an overpowering influence, there is no further essential or lasting difficulty. The choice follows upon the thought, or is simultaneous with it, and the self-consecration follows upon the choice. The feet are already set upon the path, even if they seem at first to wander uncertainly and even though the path itself may be only obscurely seen and the knowledge of the goal may be imperfect. The secret Teacher, the inner Guide is already at work, though he may not yet manifest himself or may not yet appear in the person of his human representative. Whatever difficulties and hesitations may ensue, they cannot eventually prevail against the power of the experience that has turned the current of the life. The call, once decisive, stands; the thing that has been born cannot eventually be stifled. Even if the force of circumstances prevents a regular pursuit or a full practical self-consecration from the first, still the mind has taken its bent and persists and returns with an ever-increasing effect upon its leading preoccupation. There is an ineluctable persistence of the inner being, and against it circumstances are in the end powerless, and no weakness in the nature can for long be an obstacle.

But this is not always the manner of the commencement. The sadhaka is often led gradually and there is a long space between the first turning of the mind and the full assent of the nature to the thing towards which it turns. There may at first be only a vivid intellectual interest, a forcible attraction towards the idea and some imperfect form of practice. Or perhaps there is an effort not favoured by the whole nature, a decision or a turn imposed by an intellectual influence or dictated by personal affection and admiration for someone who is himself consecrated and devoted to the Highest. In such cases, a long period of preparation may be necessary before there comes the irrevocable consecration; and in some instances it may not come. There may be some advance, there may be a strong effort, even much purification and many experiences other than those that are central or supreme; but the life will either be spent in preparation or, a certain stage having been reached, the mind pushed by an insufficient driving-force may rest content at the limit of the effort possible to it. Or there may even be a recoil to the lower life,—what is called in the ordinary parlance of Yoga a fall from the path. This lapse happens because there is a defect at the very centre. The intellect has been interested, the heart attracted, the will has strung itself to the effort, but the whole nature has not been taken captive by the Divine. It has only acquiesced in the interest, the attraction or the endeavour. There has been an experiment, perhaps even an eager experiment, but not a total self-giving to an imperative need of the soul or to an unforsakable ideal. Even such imperfect Yoga has not been wasted; for no upward effort is made in vain. Even if it fails in the present or arrives only at some preparatory stage or preliminary realisation, it has yet determined the soul's future.

But if we desire to make the most of the opportunity that this life gives us, if we wish to respond adequately to the call we have received and to attain to the goal we have glimpsed, not merely advance a little towards it, it is essential that there should be an entire self-giving. The secret of success in Yoga is to regard it not as one of the aims to be pursued in life, but as the one and only aim, not as an important part of life, but as the whole of life.

And since Yoga is in its essence a turning away from the ordinary material and animal life led by most men or from the more mental but still limited way of living followed by the few to a greater spiritual life, to the way divine, every part of our energies that is given to the lower existence in the spirit of that existence is a contradiction of our aim and our self-dedication. On the other hand, every energy or activity that we can convert from its allegiance to the lower and dedicate to the service of the higher is so much gained on our road, so much taken from the powers that oppose our progress. It is the difficulty of this wholesale conversion that is the source of all the stumblings in the path of Yoga. For our entire nature and its environment, all our personal and all our universal self, are full of habits and of influences that are opposed to our spiritual rebirth and work against the whole-heartedness of our endeavour. In a certain sense we are nothing but a complex mass of mental, nervous and physical habits held together by a few ruling ideas, desires and associations,—an amalgam of many small self-repeating forces with a few major vibrations. What we propose in our Yoga is nothing less than to break up the whole formation of our past and present which makes up the ordinary material and mental man and to create a new centre of vision and a new universe of activities in ourselves which shall constitute a divine humanity or a superhuman nature.

The first necessity is to dissolve that central faith and vision in the mind which concentrate it on its development and satisfaction and interests in the old externalised order of things. It is imperative to exchange this surface orientation for the deeper faith and vision which see only the Divine and seek only after the Divine. The next need is to compel all our lower being to pay homage to this new faith and greater vision. All our nature must make an integral surrender; it must offer itself in every part and every movement to that which seems to the unregenerated sense-mind so much less real than the material world and its objects. Our whole being—soul, mind, sense, heart, will, life, body—must consecrate all its energies so entirely and in such a way that it shall become a fit vehicle for the Divine. This is no easy task; for everything in the world follows the fixed habit which is to it a law and resists a radical change. And no change can be more radical than the revolution attempted in the integral Yoga. Everything in us has constantly to be called back to the central faith and will and vision. Every thought and impulse has to be reminded in the language of the Upanishad that "That is the divine Brahman and not this which men here adore." Every vital fibre has to be persuaded to accept an entire renunciation of all that hitherto represented to it its own existence. Mind has to cease to be mind and become brilliant with something beyond it. Life has to change into a thing vast and calm and intense and powerful that can no longer recognise its old blind eager narrow self of petty impulse and desire. Even the body has to submit to a mutation and be no longer the clamorous animal or the impeding clod it now is, but become instead a conscious servant and radiant instrument and living form of the spirit.

The difficulty of the task has led naturally to the pursuit of easy and trenchant solutions; it has generated and fixed deeply the tendency of religions and of schools of Yoga to separate the life of the world from the inner life. The powers of this world and their actual activities, it is felt, either do not belong to God at all or are for some obscure and puzzling cause, Maya or another, a dark contradiction of the divine Truth. And on their own opposite side the powers of the Truth and their ideal activities are seen to belong to quite another plane of consciousness than that, obscure, ignorant and perverse in its impulses and forces, on which the life of the earth is founded. There appears at once the antinomy of a bright and pure kingdom of God and a dark and impure kingdom of the devil; we feel the opposition of our crawling earthly birth and life to an exalted spiritual God-consciousness; we become readily convinced of the incompatibility of life's subjection to Maya with the soul's concentration in pure Brahman existence. The easiest way is to turn away from all that belongs to the one and to retreat by a naked and precipitous ascent into the other. Thus arises the attraction and, it would seem, the necessity of the principle of exclusive concentration which plays so prominent a part in the specialised schools of Yoga; for by that concentration we can arrive through an uncompromising renunciation of the world at an entire self-consecration to the One on whom we concentrate. It is no longer incumbent on us to compel all the lower activities to the difficult recognition of a new and higher spiritualised life and train them to be its agents or executive powers. It is enough to kill or quiet them and keep at most the few energies necessary, on one side, for the maintenance of the body and, on the other, for communion with the Divine.

The very aim and conception of an integral Yoga debar us from adopting this simple and strenuous high-pitched process. The hope of an integral transformation forbids us to take a short cut or to make ourselves light for the race by throwing away our impedimenta. For we have set out to conquer all ourselves and the world for God; we are determined to give him our becoming as well as our being and not merely to bring the pure and naked spirit as a bare offering to a remote and secret Divinity in a distant heaven or abolish all we are in a holocaust to an immobile Absolute. The Divine that we adore is not only a remote extra-cosmic Reality, but a half-veiled Manifestation present and near to us here in the universe. Life is the field of a divine manifestation not yet complete: here, in life, on earth, in the body,—*ihaiva*, as the Upanishads insist,—we have to unveil the Godhead; here we must make its transcendent greatness, light and sweetness real to our consciousness, here possess and, as far as may be, express it. Life then we must accept in our Yoga in order utterly to transmute it; we are forbidden to shrink from the difficulties that this acceptance may add to our struggle. Our compensation is that even if the path is more rugged, the effort more complex and bafflingly arduous, yet after a certain point we gain an immense advantage. For once our minds are reasonably fixed in the central vision and our wills are on the whole converted to the single pursuit, Life becomes our helper. Intent, vigilant, integrally conscious, we can take every detail of its forms and every incident of its movements as food for the sacrificial Fire within us. Victorious in the struggle, we can compel Earth herself to be an aid towards our perfection and can enrich our realisation with the booty torn from the Powers that oppose us.

There is another direction in which the ordinary practice of Yoga arrives at a helpful but narrowing simplification which is denied to the sadhaka of the integral aim. The practice of Yoga brings us face to face with the extraordinary complexity of our own being, the stimulating but also embarrassing multiplicity of our personality, the rich endless confusion of Nature. To the ordinary man who lives upon his own waking surface, ignorant of the self's depths and vastnesses behind the veil, his psychological existence is fairly simple. A small but clamorous company of desires, some imperative intellectual and aesthetic cravings, some tastes, a few ruling or prominent ideas amid a great current of unconnected or ill-connected and mostly trivial thoughts, a number of more or less imperative vital needs, alternations of physical health and disease, a scattered and inconsequent succession of joys and griefs, frequent minor disturbances and vicissitudes and rarer strong searchings and upheavals of mind or body, and through it all Nature, partly with the aid of his thought and will, partly without or in spite of it, arranging these things in some rough practical fashion, some tolerable disorderly order,—this is the material of his existence. The average human being even now is in his inward existence as crude and undeveloped as was the bygone primitive man in his outward life. But as soon as we go deep within ourselves,—and Yoga means a plunge into all the multiple profundities of the soul,—we find ourselves subjectively, as man in his growth has found himself objectively, surrounded by a whole complex world which we have to know and to conquer.

The most disconcerting discovery is to find that every part of us—intellect, will, sense-mind, nervous or desire self, the heart, the body—has each, as it were, its own complex individuality and natural formation independent of the rest; it neither agrees with itself nor with the others nor with the representative ego which is the shadow cast by some central and centralising self on our superficial ignorance. We find that we are composed not of one but many personalities and each has its own demands and differing nature. Our being is a roughly constituted chaos into which we have to introduce the principle of a divine order. Moreover, we find that inwardly too, no less than outwardly, we are not alone in the world; the sharp separateness of our ego was no more than a strong imposition and delusion; we do not exist in ourselves, we do not really live apart in an inner privacy or solitude. Our mind is a receiving, developing and modifying machine into which there is being constantly passed from moment to moment a ceaseless foreign flux, a streaming mass of disparate materials from above, from below, from outside. Much more than half our thoughts and feelings are not our own in the sense that they take form out of ourselves; of hardly anything can it be said that it is truly original to our nature. A large part comes to us from others or from the environment, whether as raw material or as manufactured imports; but still more largely they come from universal Nature here or from other worlds and planes and their beings and powers and influences; for we are overtopped and environed by other planes of consciousness, mind planes, life planes, subtle matter planes, from which our life and action here are fed, or fed on, pressed, dominated, made use of for the manifestation of their forms and forces. The difficulty of our separate salvation is immensely increased by this complexity and manifold openness and subjection to the in-streaming energies of the universe. Of all this we have to take account, to deal with it, to know what is the secret stuff of our nature and its constituent and resultant motions and to create in it all a divine centre and a true harmony and luminous order.

In the ordinary paths of Yoga the method used for dealing with these conflicting materials is direct and simple. One or another of the principal psychological forces in us is selected as our single means for attaining to the Divine; the rest is quieted into inertia or left to starve in its smallness. The Bhakta, seizing on the emotional forces of the being, the intense activities of the heart, abides concentrated in the love of God, gathered up as into a single one-pointed tongue of fire; he is indifferent to the activities of thought, throws behind him the importunities of the reason, cares nothing for the mind's thirst for knowledge. All the knowledge he needs is his faith and the inspirations that well up from a heart in communion with the Divine. He has no use for any will to works that is not turned to the direct worship of the Beloved or the service of the temple. The man of Knowledge, self-confined by a deliberate choice to the force and activities of discriminative thought, finds release in the mind's hushed inward-drawn endeavour. He concentrates on the idea of the self, succeeds by a subtle inner discernment in distinguishing its silent presence amid the veiling activities of Nature, and through the perceptive idea arrives at the concrete spiritual experience. He is indifferent to the play of the emotions, deaf to the hunger-call of passion, closed to the activities of Life,—the more blessed he, the sooner they fall away from him and leave him free, still and mute, the eternal non-doer. The body is his stumbling-block, the vital functions are his enemies; if their demands can be reduced to a minimum, that is his great good fortune. The endless difficulties that arise from the environing world are dismissed by erecting firmly against them a defence of outer physical and inner spiritual solitude; safe behind a wall of inner silence, he remains impassive and untouched by the world and by others. To be alone with oneself or alone with the Divine, to walk apart with God and his devotees, to entrench oneself in the single self-ward endeavour of the mind or Godward passion of the heart is the trend of these Yogas. The problem is solved by the excision of all but the one central difficulty which pursues the one chosen motive-force; into the midst of the dividing calls of our nature the principle of an exclusive concentration comes sovereignly to our rescue.

But for the sadhaka of the integral Yoga this inner or this outer solitude can only be incidents or periods in his spiritual progress. Accepting life, he has to bear not only his own burden, but a great part of the world's burden too along with it, as a continuation of his own sufficiently heavy load. Therefore his Yoga has much more of the nature of a battle than others; but this is not only an individual battle, it is a collective war waged over a considerable country. He has not only to conquer in himself the forces of egoistic falsehood and disorder, but to conquer them as representatives of the same adverse and inexhaustible forces in the world. Their representative character gives them a much more obstinate capacity of resistance, an almost endless right to recurrence. Often he finds that even after he has won persistently his own personal battle, he has still to win it over and over again in a seemingly interminable war, because his inner existence has already been so much enlarged that not only it contains his own being with its well-defined needs and experiences, but is in solidarity with the being of others, because in himself he contains the universe.

Nor is the seeker of the integral fulfilment permitted to solve too arbitrarily even the conflict of his own inner members. He has to harmonise deliberate knowledge with unquestioning faith; he must conciliate the gentle soul of love with the formidable need of power; the passivity of the soul that lives content in transcendent calm has to be fused with the activity of the divine helper and the divine warrior. To him as to all seekers of the spirit there are offered for solution the oppositions of the reason, the clinging hold of the senses, the perturbations of the heart, the ambush of the desires, the clog of the physical body; but he has to deal in another fashion with their mutual and internal conflicts and their hindrance to his aim, for he must arrive at an infinitely more difficult perfection in the handling of all this rebel matter. Accepting them as instruments for the divine realisation and manifestation, he has to convert their jangling discords, to enlighten their thick darknesses, to transfigure them separately and all together, harmonising them in themselves and with each other,—integrally, omitting no grain or strand or vibration, leaving no iota of imperfection anywhere. An exclusive concentration, or even a succession of concentrations of that kind, can be in his complex work only a temporary convenience; it has to be abandoned as soon as its utility is over. An all-inclusive concentration is the difficult achievement towards which he must labour.

Concentration is indeed the first condition of any Yoga, but it is an all-receiving concentration that is the very nature of the integral Yoga. A separate strong fixing of the thought, of the emotions or of the will on a single idea, object, state, inner movement or principle is no doubt a frequent need here also; but this is only a subsidiary helpful process. A wide massive opening, a harmonised concentration of the whole being in all its parts and through all its powers upon the One who is the All is the larger action of this Yoga without which it cannot achieve its purpose. For it is the consciousness that rests in the One and that acts in the All to which we aspire; it is this that we seek to impose on every element of our being and on every movement of our nature. This wide and concentrated totality is the essential character of the Sadhana and its character must determine its practice.

But even though the concentration of all the being on the Divine is the character of the Yoga, yet is our being too complex a thing to be taken up easily and at once, as if we were taking up the world in a pair of hands, and set in its entirety to a single task. Man in his effort at self-transcendence has usually to seize on some one spring or some powerful leverage in the complicated machine that his nature is; this spring or lever he touches in preference to others and uses it to set the machine in motion towards the end that he has in view. In his choice it is always Nature itself that should be his guide. But here it must be Nature at her highest and widest in him, not at her lowest or in some limiting movement. In her lower vital activities it is desire that Nature takes as her most powerful leverage; but the distinct character of man is that he is a mental being, not a merely vital creature. As he can use his thinking mind and will to restrain and correct his life impulses, so too he can bring in the action of a still higher luminous mentality aided by the deeper soul in him, the psychic being, and supersede by these greater and purer motive-powers the domination of the vital and sensational force that we call desire. He can entirely master or persuade it and offer it up for transformation to its divine Master. This higher mentality and this deeper soul, the psychic element in man, are the two grappling hooks by which the Divine can lay hold upon his nature.

The higher mind in man is something other, loftier, purer, vaster, more powerful than the reason or logical intelligence. The animal is a vital and sensational being; man, it is said, is distinguished from the animal by the possession of reason. But that is a very summary, a very imperfect and misleading account of the matter. For reason is only a particular and limited utilitarian and instrumental activity that proceeds from something much greater than itself, from a power that dwells in an ether more luminous, wider, illimitable. The true and ultimate, as distinguished from the immediate or intermediate importance of our observing, reasoning, inquiring, judging intelligence is that it prepares the human being for the right reception and right action of a Light from above which must progressively replace in him the obscure light from below that guides the animal. The latter also has a rudimentary reason, a kind of thought, a soul, a will and keen emotions; even though less developed, its psychology is yet the same in kind as man's. But all these capacities in the animal are automatically moved and strictly limited, almost even constituted by the lower nervous being. All animal perceptions, sensibilities, activities are ruled by nervous and vital instincts, cravings, needs, satisfactions, of which the nexus is the life-impulse and vital desire. Man too is bound, but less bound, to this automatism of the vital nature. Man can bring an enlightened will, an enlightened thought and enlightened emotions to the difficult work of his self-development; he can more and more subject to these more conscious and reflecting guides the inferior function of desire. In proportion as he can thus master and enlighten his lower self, he is man and no longer an animal. When he can begin to replace desire altogether by a still greater enlightened thought and sight and will in touch with the Infinite, consciously subject to a diviner will than his own, linked to a more universal and transcendent knowledge, he has commenced the ascent towards the superman; he is on his upward march towards the Divine.

It is, then, in the highest mind of thought and light and will or it is in the inner heart of deepest feeling and emotion that we must first centre our consciousness,—in either of them or, if we are capable, in both together,—

and use that as our leverage to lift the nature wholly towards the Divine. The concentration of an enlightened thought, will and heart turned in unison towards one vast goal of our knowledge, one luminous and infinite source of our action, one imperishable object of our emotion is the starting-point of the Yoga. And the object of our seeking must be the very fount of the Light which is growing in us, the very origin of the Force which we are calling to move our members. Our one objective must be the Divine himself to whom, knowingly or unknowingly, something always aspires in our secret nature. There must be a large, many-sided yet single concentration of the thought on the idea, the perception, the vision, the awakening touch, the soul's realisation of the one Divine. There must be a flaming concentration of the heart on the seeking of the All and Eternal and, when once we have found him, a deep plunging and immersion in the possession and ecstasy of the All-Beautiful. There must be a strong and immovable concentration of the will on the attainment and fulfilment of all that the Divine is and a free and plastic opening of it to all that he intends to manifest in us. This is the triple way of the Yoga.

But on that which as yet we know not how shall we concentrate? And yet we cannot know the Divine unless we have achieved this concentration of our being upon him. A concentration which culminates in a living realisation and the constant sense of the presence of the One in ourselves and in all of which we are aware, is what we mean in Yoga by knowledge and the effort after knowledge. It is not enough to devote ourselves by the reading of Scriptures or by the stress of philosophic reasoning to an intellectual understanding of the Divine; for at the end of our long mental labour we might know all that has been said of the Eternal, possess all that can be thought about the Infinite and yet we might not know him at all. This intellectual preparation can indeed be the first stage in a powerful Yoga, but it is not indispensable: it is not a step which all need or can be called upon to take. Yoga would be impossible, except for a very few, if the intellectual figure of knowledge arrived at by the speculative or meditative Reason were its indispensable condition or a binding preliminary. All that the Light from above asks of us that it may begin its work is a call from the soul and a sufficient point of support in the mind. This support can be reached through an insistent idea of the Divine in the thought, a corresponding will in the dynamic parts, an aspiration, a faith, a need in the heart. Any one of these may lead or predominate, if all cannot move in unison or in an equal rhythm. The idea may be and must in the beginning be inadequate; the aspiration may be narrow and imperfect, the faith poorly illumined or even, as not surely founded on the rock of knowledge, fluctuating, uncertain, easily diminished; often even it may be extinguished and need to be lit again with difficulty like a torch in a windy pass. But if once there is a resolute self-consecration from deep within, if there is an awakening to the soul's call, these inadequate things can be a sufficient instrument for the divine purpose. Therefore the wise have always been unwilling to limit man's avenues towards God; they would not shut against his entry even the narrowest portal, the lowest and darkest postern, the humblest wicket-gate. Any name, any form, any symbol, any offering has been held to be sufficient if there is the consecration along with it; for the Divine knows himself in the heart of the seeker and accepts the sacrifice.

But still the greater and wider the moving idea-force behind the consecration, the better for the seeker; his attainment is likely to be fuller and more ample. If we are to attempt an integral Yoga, it will be as well to start with an idea of the Divine that is itself integral. There should be an aspiration in the heart wide enough for a realisation without any narrow limits. Not only should we avoid a sectarian religious outlook, but also all one-sided philosophical conceptions which try to shut up the Ineffable in a restricting mental formula. The dynamic conception or impelling sense with which our Yoga can best set out would be naturally the idea, the sense of a conscious all-embracing but all-exceeding Infinite. Our up-look must be to a free, all-powerful, perfect and blissful One and Oneness in which all beings move and live and through which all can meet and become one. This Eternal will be at once personal and impersonal in his self-revelation and touch upon the soul. He is personal because he is the conscious Divine, the infinite Person who casts some broken reflection of himself in the myriad divine and undivine personalities of the universe. He is impersonal because he appears to us as an infinite Existence, Consciousness and Ananda and because he is the fount, base and constituent of all existences and all energies, the very material of our being and mind and life and body, our spirit and our matter. The thought, concentrating on him, must not merely understand in an intellectual form that he exists, or conceive of him as an abstraction, a logical necessity; it must become a seeing thought able to meet him here as the Inhabitant in all, realise him in ourselves, watch and take hold on the movement of his forces. He is the one Existence: he is the original and universal Delight that constitutes all things and exceeds them: he is the one infinite Consciousness that composes all consciousnesses and informs all their movements: he is the one illimitable Being who sustains all action and experience: his will guides the evolution of things towards their yet unrealised but inevitable aim and plenitude. To him the heart can consecrate itself, approach him as the supreme Beloved, beat and move in him as in a universal sweetness of Love and a living sea of Delight. For his is the secret Joy that supports the soul in all its experiences and maintains even the errant ego in its ordeals and struggles till all sorrow and suffering shall cease. His is the Love and the Bliss of the infinite divine Lover who is drawing all things by their own path towards his happy oneness. On him the Will can unalterably fix as the invisible Power that guides and fulfils it and as the source of its strength. In the impersonality this actuating Power is a self-illumined Force that contains all results and calmly works until it accomplishes, in the personality an all-wise and omnipotent Master of the Yoga whom nothing can prevent from leading it to its goal. This is the faith with which the seeker has to begin his seeking and endeavour; for in all his effort here, but most of all in his effort towards the Unseen, mental man must perforce proceed by faith. When the realisation comes, the faith divinely fulfilled and completed will be transformed into an eternal flame of knowledge.

Into all our endeavour upward the lower element of desire will at first naturally enter. For what the enlightened will sees as the thing to be done and pursues as the crown to be conquered, what the heart embraces as the one thing delightful, that in us which feels itself limited and opposed and, because it is limited, craves and struggles, will seek with the troubled passion of an egoistic desire. This craving life-force or desire-soul in us has to be accepted at first, but only in order that it may be transformed. Even from the very beginning it has to be taught to renounce all other desires and concentrate itself on the passion for the Divine. This capital point gained, it has to be taught to desire, not for its own separate sake, but for God in the world and for the Divine in ourselves; it has to fix itself upon no personal spiritual gain, though of all possible spiritual gains we are sure, but on the great work to be done in us and others, on the high coming manifestation which is to be the glorious fulfilment of the Divine in the world, on the Truth that has to be sought and lived and enthroned for ever. But last, most difficult for it, more difficult than to seek with the right object, it has to be taught to seek in the right manner; for it must learn to desire, not in its own egoistic way, but in the way of the Divine. It must insist no longer, as the strong separative will always insists, on its own manner of fulfilment, its own dream of possession, its own idea of the right and the desirable; it must yearn to fulfil a larger and greater Will and consent to wait upon a less interested and ignorant guidance. Thus trained, Desire, that great unquiet harasser and troubler of man and cause of every kind of stumbling, will become fit to be transformed into its divine counterpart. For desire and passion too have their divine forms; there is a pure ecstasy of the soul's seeking beyond all craving and grief, there is a Will of Ananda that sits glorified in the possession of the supreme beatitudes.

When once the object of concentration has possessed and is possessed by the three master instruments, the thought, the heart and the will,—a consummation fully possible only when the desire-soul in us has submitted to the Divine Law,—the perfection of mind and life and body can be effectively fulfilled in our transmuted nature. This will be done, not for the personal satisfaction of the ego, but that the whole may constitute a fit temple for the Divine Presence, a faultless instrument for the divine work. For that work can be truly performed only when the instrument, consecrated and perfected, has grown fit for a selfless action,—and that will be when personal desire and egoism are abolished, but not the liberated individual. Even when the little ego has been abolished, the true spiritual Person can still remain and God's will and work and delight in him and the spiritual use of his perfection and fulfilment. Our works will then be divine and done divinely; our mind and life and will, devoted to the Divine, will be used to help fulfil in others and in the world that which has been first realised in ourselves,—all that we can manifest of the embodied Unity, Love, Freedom, Strength, Power, Splendour, immortal Joy which is the goal of the Spirit's terrestrial adventure.

The Yoga must start with an effort or at least a settled turn towards this total concentration. A constant and unfailing will of consecration of all ourselves to the Supreme is demanded of us, an offering of our whole being and our many-chambered nature to the Eternal who is the All. The effective fullness of our concentration on the one thing needful to the exclusion of all else will be the measure of our self-consecration to the One who is alone desirable. But this exclusiveness will in the end exclude nothing except the falsehood of our way of seeing the world and our will's ignorance. For our concentration on the Eternal will be consummated by the mind when we see constantly the Divine in itself and the Divine in ourselves, but also the Divine in all things and beings and happenings. It will be consummated by the heart when all emotion is summed up in the love of the Divine,—of the Divine in itself and for itself, but love too of the Divine in all its beings and powers and personalities and forms in the Universe. It will be consummated by the will when we feel and receive always the divine impulsion and accept that alone as our sole motive force; but this will mean that, having slain to the last rebellious straggler the wandering impulses of the egoistic nature, we have universalised ourselves and can accept with a constant happy acceptance the one divine working in all things. This is the first fundamental siddhi of the integral Yoga.

It is nothing less that is meant in the end when we speak of the absolute consecration of the individual to the Divine. But this total fullness of consecration can only come by a constant progression when the long and difficult process of transforming desire out of existence is completed in an ungrudging measure. Perfect self-consecration implies perfect self-surrender.

For here, there are two movements with a transitional stage between them, two periods of this Yoga,—one of the process of surrender, the other of its crown and consequence. In the first the individual prepares himself for the reception of the Divine into his members. For all this first period he has to work by means of the instruments of the lower Nature, but aided more and more from above. But in the later transitional stage of this movement our personal and necessarily ignorant effort more and more dwindles and a higher Nature acts; the eternal Shakti descends into this limited form of mortality and progressively possesses and transmutes it. In the second period the greater movement wholly replaces the lesser, formerly indispensable first action; but this can be done only when our self-surrender is complete. The ego person in us cannot transform itself by its own force or will or knowledge or by any virtue of its own into the nature of the Divine; all it can do is to fit itself for the transformation and make more and more its surrender to that which it seeks to become. As long as the ego is at work in us, our personal action is and must always be in its nature a part of the lower grades of existence; it is obscure or half-enlightened, limited in its field, very partially effective in its power. If a spiritual transformation, not a mere illumining modification of our nature, is to be done at all, we must call in the Divine Shakti to effect that miraculous work in the individual; for she alone has the needed force, decisive, all-wise and illimitable. But the entire substitution of the divine for the human personal action is not at once entirely possible.

All interference from below that would falsify the truth of the superior action must first be inhibited or rendered impotent, and it must be done by our own free choice. A continual and always repeated refusal of the impulsions and falsehoods of the lower nature is asked from us and an insistent support to the Truth as it grows in our parts; for the progressive settling into our nature and final perfection of the incoming informing Light, Purity and Power needs for its development and sustenance our free acceptance of it and our stubborn rejection of all that is contrary to it, inferior or incompatible.

In the first movement of self-preparation, the period of personal effort, the method we have to use is this concentration of the whole being on the Divine that it seeks and, as its corollary, this constant rejection, throwing out, *katharsis*, of all that is not the true Truth of the Divine. An entire consecration of all that we are, think, feel and do will be the result of this persistence. This consecration in its turn must culminate in an integral self-giving to the Highest; for its crown and sign of completion is the whole nature's all-comprehending absolute surrender. In the second stage of the Yoga, transitional between the human and the divine working, there will supervene an increasing purified and vigilant passivity, a more and more luminous divine response to the Divine Force, but not to any other; and there will be as a result the growing inrush of a great and conscious miraculous working from above. In the last period there is no effort at all, no set method, no fixed sadhana; the place of endeavour and tapasya will be taken by a natural, simple, powerful and happy disclosing of the flower of the Divine out of the bud of a purified and perfected terrestrial nature. These are the natural successions of the action of the Yoga.

These movements are indeed not always or absolutely arranged in a strict succession to each other. The second stage begins in part before the first is completed; the first continues in part until the second is perfected; the last divine working can manifest from time to time as a promise before it is finally settled and normal to the nature. Always too there is something higher and greater than the individual which leads him even in his personal labour and endeavour. Often he may become, and remain for a time, wholly conscious, even in parts of his being permanently conscious, of this greater leading behind the veil, and that may happen long before his whole nature has been purified in all its parts from the lower indirect control. Even, he may be thus conscious from the beginning; his mind and heart, if not his other members, may respond to that seizing and penetrating guidance with a certain initial completeness from the very first steps of the Yoga. But it is the constant and complete and uniform action of the great direct control that more and more distinguishes the transitional stage as it proceeds and draws to its close. This predominance of a greater diviner leading, not personal to ourselves, indicates the nature's increasing ripeness for a total spiritual transformation. It is the unmistakable sign that the self-consecration has not only been accepted in principle but is fulfilled in act and power. The Supreme has laid his luminous hand upon a chosen human vessel of his miraculous Light and Power and Ananda.

CHAPTER III. SELF-SURRENDER IN WORKS — THE WAY OF THE GITA

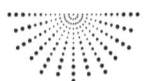

LIFE, NOT a remote silent or high-uplifted ecstatic Beyond Life alone, is the field of our Yoga. The transformation of our superficial, narrow and fragmentary human way of thinking, seeing, feeling and being into a deep and wide spiritual consciousness and an integrated inner and outer existence and of our ordinary human living into the divine way of life must be its central purpose. The means towards this supreme end is a self-giving of all our nature to the Divine. Everything must be given to the Divine within us, to the universal All and to the transcendent Supreme. An absolute concentration of our will, our heart and our thought on that one and manifold Divine, an unreserved self-consecration of our whole being to the Divine alone—this is the decisive movement, the turning of the ego to That which is infinitely greater than itself, its self-giving and indispensable surrender.

The life of the human creature, as it is ordinarily lived, is composed of a half-fixed, half-fluid mass of very imperfectly ruled thoughts, perceptions, sensations, emotions, desires, enjoyments, acts, mostly customary and self-repeating, in part only dynamic and self-developing, but all centred around a superficial ego. The sum of movement of these activities eventuates in an internal growth which is partly visible and operative in this life, partly a seed of progress in lives hereafter. This growth of the conscious being, an expansion, an increasing self-expression, a more and more harmonised development of his constituent members is the whole meaning and all the pith of human existence. It is for this meaningful development of consciousness by thought, will, emotion, desire, action and experience, leading in the end to a supreme divine self-discovery, that Man, the mental being, has entered into the material body. All the rest is either auxiliary and subordinate or accidental and otiose; that only matters which sustains and helps the evolution of his nature and the growth or rather the progressive unfolding and discovery of his self and spirit.

The aim set before our Yoga is nothing less than to hasten this supreme object of our existence here. Its process leaves behind the ordinary tardy method of slow and confused growth through the evolution of Nature. For the natural evolution is at its best an uncertain growth under cover, partly by the pressure of the environment, partly by a groping education and an ill-lighted purposeful effort, an only partially illumined and half-automatic use of opportunities with many blunders and lapses and relapses; a great portion of it is made up of apparent accidents and circumstances and vicissitudes,—though veiling a secret divine intervention and guidance. In Yoga we replace this confused crooked crab-motion by a rapid, conscious and self-directed evolution which is planned to carry us, as far as can be, in a straight line towards the goal set before us. In a certain sense it may be an error to speak of a goal anywhere in a progression which may well be infinite. Still we can conceive of an immediate goal, an ulterior objective beyond our present achievement towards which the soul in man can aspire. There lies before him the possibility of a new birth; there can be an ascent into a higher and wider plane of being and its descent to transform his members. An enlarged and illumined consciousness is possible that shall make of him a liberated spirit and a perfected force—and, if spread beyond the individual, it might even constitute a divine humanity or else a new, a supramental and therefore a superhuman race. It is this new birth that we make our aim: a growth into a divine consciousness is the whole meaning of our Yoga, an integral conversion to divinity not only of the soul but of all the parts of our nature.

~

Our purpose in Yoga is to exile the limited outward-looking ego and to enthrone God in its place as the ruling Inhabitant of the nature. And this means, first, to disinherit desire and no longer accept the enjoyment of desire as the ruling human motive. The spiritual life will draw its sustenance not from desire but from a pure and selfless spiritual delight of essential existence. And not only the vital nature in us whose stamp is desire, but the mental being too must undergo a new birth and a transfiguring change. Our divided, egoistic, limited and ignorant thought and intelligence must disappear; in its place there must stream in the catholic and faultless play of a shadowless divine illumination which shall culminate in the end in a natural self-existent Truth-consciousness free from groping half-truth and stumbling error. Our confused and embarrassed ego-centred small-motived will and action must cease and make room for the total working of a swiftly powerful, lucidly automatic, divinely moved and guided unfallen Force. There must be implanted and activised in all our doings a supreme, impersonal, unfaltering and unstumbling will in spontaneous and untroubled unison with the will of the Divine. The unsatisfying surface play of our feeble egoistic emotions must be ousted and there must be revealed instead a secret deep and vast psychic heart within that waits behind them for its hour; all our feelings, impelled by this inner heart in which dwells the Divine, will be transmuted into calm and intense movements of a twin passion of divine Love and manifold Ananda. This is the definition of a divine humanity or a supramental race. This, not an exaggerated or even a sublimated energy of human intellect and action, is the type of the superman whom we are called to evolve by our Yoga.

In the ordinary human existence an outgoing action is obviously three-fourths or even more of our life. It is only the exceptions, the saint and the seer, the rare thinker, poet and artist who can live more within themselves; these indeed, at least in the most intimate parts of their nature, shape themselves more in inner thought and feeling than in the surface act. But it is not either of these sides separated from the other, but rather a harmony of the inner and the outer life made one in fullness and transfigured into a play of something that is beyond them which will create the form of a perfect living. A Yoga of works, a union with the Divine in our will and acts—and not only in knowledge and feeling—is then an indispensable, an inexpressibly important element of an integral Yoga. The conversion of our thought and feeling without a corresponding conversion of the spirit and body of our works would be a maimed achievement.

But if this total conversion is to be done, there must be a consecration of our actions and outer movements as much as of our mind and heart to the Divine. There must be accepted and progressively accomplished a surrender of our capacities of working into the hands of a greater Power behind us and our sense of being the doer and worker must disappear. All must be given for a more direct use into the hands of the divine Will which is hidden by these frontal appearances; for by that permitting Will alone is our action possible. A hidden Power is the true Lord and overruling Observer of our acts and only he knows through all the ignorance and perversion and deformation brought in by the ego their entire sense and ultimate purpose. There must be effected a complete transformation of our limited and distorted egoistic life and works into the large and direct outpouring of a greater divine Life, Will and Energy that now secretly supports us. This greater Will and Energy must be made conscious in us and master; no longer must it remain, as now, only a superconscious, upholding and permitting Force. There must be achieved an undistorted transmission through us of the all-wise purpose and process of a now hidden omniscient Power and omnipotent Knowledge which will turn into its pure, unobstructed, happily consenting and participating channel all our transmuted nature. This total consecration and surrender and this resultant entire transformation and free transmission make up the whole fundamental means and the ultimate aim of an integral Karmayoga.

Even for those whose first natural movement is a consecration, a surrender and a resultant entire transformation of the thinking mind and its knowledge, or a total consecration, surrender and transformation of the heart and its emotions, the consecration of works is a needed element in that change. Otherwise, although they may find God in other-life, they will not be able to fulfil the Divine in life; life for them will be a meaningless undivine inconsequence. Not for them the true victory that shall be the key to the riddle of our terrestrial existence; their love will not be the absolute love triumphant over self, their knowledge will not be the total consciousness and the all-embracing knowledge. It is possible, indeed, to begin with knowledge or Godward emotion solely or with both together and to leave works for the final movement of the Yoga. But there is then this disadvantage that we may tend to live too exclusively within, subtilised in subjective experience, shut off in our isolated inner parts; there we may get incrusted in our spiritual seclusion and find it difficult later on to pour ourselves triumphantly outwards and apply to life our gains in the higher Nature. When we turn to add this external kingdom also to our inner conquests, we shall find ourselves too much accustomed to an activity purely subjective and ineffective on the material plane. There will be an immense difficulty in transforming the outer life and the body. Or we shall find that our action does not correspond with the inner light: it still follows the old accustomed mistaken paths, still obeys the old normal imperfect influences; the Truth within us continues to be separated by a painful gulf from the ignorant mechanism of our external nature. This is a frequent experience because in such a process the Light and Power come to be self-contained and unwilling to express themselves in life or to use the physical means prescribed for the Earth and her processes. It is as if we were living in another, a larger and subtler world and had no divine hold, perhaps little hold of any kind, upon the material and terrestrial existence.

But still each must follow his nature, and there are always difficulties that have to be accepted for some time if we are to pursue our natural path of Yoga. Yoga is after all primarily a change of the inner consciousness and nature, and if the balance of our parts is such that this must be done first with an initial exclusiveness and the rest left for later handling, we must accept the apparent imperfection of the process. Yet would the ideal working of an integral Yoga be a movement, even from the beginning, integral in its process and whole and many-sided in its progress. In any case our present preoccupation is with a Yoga, integral in its aim and complete movement, but starting from works and proceeding by works although at each step more and more moved by a vivifying divine love and more and more illumined by a helping divine knowledge.

The greatest gospel of spiritual works ever yet given to the race, the most perfect system of Karmayoga known to man in the past, is to be found in the Bhagavad Gita. In that famous episode of the Mahabharata the great basic lines of Karmayoga are laid down for all time with an incomparable mastery and the infallible eye of an assured experience. It is true that the path alone, as the ancients saw it, is worked out fully: the perfect fulfilment, the highest secret[1] is hinted rather than developed; it is kept back as an unexpressed part of a supreme mystery. There are obvious reasons for this reticence; for the fulfilment is in any case a matter for experience and no teaching can express it. It cannot be described in a way that can really be understood by a mind that has not the effulgent transmuting experience. And for the soul that has passed the shining portals and stands in the blaze of the inner light, all mental and verbal description is as poor as it is superfluous, inadequate and an impertinence. All divine consummations have perforce to be figured by us in the inapt and deceptive terms of a language which was made to fit the normal experience of mental man; so expressed, they can be rightly understood only by those who already know, and, knowing, are able to give these poor external terms a changed, inner and transfigured sense. As the Vedic Rishis insisted in the beginning, the words of the supreme wisdom are expressive only to those who are already of the wise. The Gita at its cryptic close may seem by its silence to stop short of that solution for which we are seeking; it pauses at the borders of the highest spiritual mind and does not cross them into the splendours of the supramental Light. And yet its secret of dynamic, and not only static, identity with the inner Presence, its highest mystery of absolute surrender to the Divine Guide, Lord and Inhabitant of our nature, is the central secret. This surrender is the indispensable means of the supramental change and, again, it is through the supramental change that the dynamic identity becomes possible.

What then are the lines of Karmayoga laid down by the Gita? Its key principle, its spiritual method, can be summed up as the union of two largest and highest states or powers of consciousness, equality and oneness. The kernel of its method is an unreserved acceptance of the Divine in our life as in our inner self and spirit. An inner renunciation of personal desire leads to equality, accomplishes our total surrender to the Divine, supports a delivery from dividing ego which brings us oneness. But this must be a oneness in dynamic force and not only in static peace or inactive beatitude. The Gita promises us freedom for the spirit even in the midst of works and the full energies of Nature, if we accept subjection of our whole being to that which is higher than the separating and limiting ego. It proposes an integral dynamic activity founded on a still passivity; a largest possible action irrevocably based on an immobile calm is its secret, —free expression out of a supreme inward silence.

All things here are the one and indivisible eternal transcendent and cosmic Brahman that is in its seeming divided in things and creatures; in seeming only, for in truth it is always one and equal in all things and creatures and the division is only a phenomenon of the surface. As long as we live in the ignorant seeming, we are the ego and are subject to the modes of Nature. Enslaved to appearances, bound to the dualities, tossed between good and evil, sin and virtue, grief and joy, pain and pleasure, good fortune and ill fortune, success and failure, we follow helplessly the iron or gilt and iron round of the wheel of Maya. At best we have only the poor relative freedom which by us is ignorantly called free-will. But that is at bottom illusory, since it is the modes of Nature that express themselves through our personal will; it is force of Nature, grasping us, ungrasped by us that determines what we shall will and how we shall will it. Nature, not an independent ego, chooses what object we shall seek, whether by reasoned will or unreflecting impulse, at any moment of our existence. If, on the contrary, we live in the unifying reality of the Brahman, then we go beyond the ego and overstep Nature. For then we get back to our true self and become the spirit; in the spirit we are above the impulsion of Nature, superior to her modes and forces. Attaining to a perfect equality in the soul, mind and heart, we realise our true self of oneness, one with all beings, one too with That which expresses itself in them and in all that we see and experience. This equality and this oneness are the indispensable twin foundation we must lay down for a divine being, a divine consciousness, a divine action. Not one with all, we are not spiritual, not divine. Not equal-souled to all things, happenings and creatures, we cannot see spiritually, cannot know divinely, cannot feel divinely towards others. The Supreme Power, the one Eternal and Infinite is equal to all things and to all beings; and because it is equal, it can act with an absolute wisdom according to the truth of its works and its force and according to the truth of each thing and of every creature.

This is also the only true freedom possible to man,—a freedom which he cannot have unless he outgrows his mental separativeness and becomes the conscious soul in Nature. The only free will in the world is the one divine Will of which Nature is the executrix; for she is the master and creator of all other wills. Human free-will can be real in a sense, but, like all things that belong to the modes of Nature, it is only relatively real. The mind rides on a swirl of natural forces, balances on a poise between several possibilities, inclines to one side or another, settles and has the sense of choosing: but it does not see, it is not even dimly aware of the Force behind that has determined its choice. It cannot see it, because that Force is something total and to our eyes indeterminate. At most mind can only distinguish with an approach to clarity and precision some out of the complex variety of particular determinations by which this Force works out her incalculable purposes. Partial itself, the mind rides on a part of the machine, unaware of nine-tenths of its motor agencies in Time and environment, unaware of its past preparation and future drift; but because it rides, it thinks that it is directing the machine. In a sense it counts: for that clear inclination of the mind which we call our will, that firm settling of the inclination which presents itself to us as a deliberate choice, is one of Nature's most powerful determinants; but it is never independent and sole. Behind this petty instrumental action of the human will there is something vast and powerful and eternal that oversees the trend of the inclination and presses on the turn of the will. There is a total Truth in Nature greater than our individual choice. And in this total Truth, or even beyond and behind it, there is something that determines all results; its presence and secret knowledge keep up steadily in the process of Nature a dynamic, almost automatic perception of the right relations, the varying or persistent necessities, the inevitable steps of the movement. There is a secret divine Will, eternal and infinite, omniscient and omnipotent, that expresses itself in the universality and in each particular of all these apparently temporal and finite inconscient or half-conscient things. This is the Power or Presence meant by the Gita when it speaks of the Lord within the heart of all existences who turns all creatures as if mounted on a machine by the illusion of Nature.

This divine Will is not an alien Power or Presence; it is intimate to us and we ourselves are part of it: for it is our own highest Self that possesses and supports it. Only, it is not our conscious mental will; it rejects often enough what our conscious will accepts and accepts what our conscious will rejects. For while this secret One knows all and every whole and each detail, our surface mind knows only a little part of things. Our will is conscious in the mind, and what it knows, it knows by the thought only; the divine Will is superconscious to us because it is in its essence supramental, and it knows all because it is all. Our highest Self which possesses and supports this universal Power is not our ego-self, not our personal nature; it is something transcendent and universal of which these smaller things are only foam and flowing surface. If we surrender our conscious will and allow it to be made one with the will of the Eternal, then, and then only, shall we attain to a true freedom; living in the divine liberty, we shall no longer cling to this shackled so-called freewill, a puppet freedom ignorant, illusory, relative, bound to the error of its own inadequate vital motives and mental figures.

∼

A distinction has to be firmly seized in our consciousness, the capital distinction between mechanical Nature and the free Lord of Nature, between the Ishwara or single luminous divine Will and the many executive modes and forces of the universe.

Nature,—not as she is in her divine Truth, the conscious Power of the Eternal, but as she appears to us in the Ignorance,—is executive Force, mechanical in her steps, not consciously intelligent to our experience of her, although all her works are instinct with an absolute intelligence. Not in herself master, she is full of a self-aware Power[2] which has an infinite mastery and, because of this Power driving her, she rules all and exactly fulfils the work intended in her by the Ishwara. Not enjoying but enjoyed, she bears in herself the burden of all enjoyments. Nature as Prakriti is an inertly active Force,—for she works out a movement imposed upon her; but within her is One that knows,—some Entity sits there that is aware of all her motion and process. Prakriti works containing the knowledge, the mastery, the delight of the Purusha, the Being associated with her or seated within her; but she can participate in them only by subjection and reflection of that which fills her. Purusha knows and is still and inactive; he contains the action of Prakriti within his consciousness and knowledge and enjoys it. He gives the sanction to Prakriti's works and she works out what is sanctioned by him for his pleasure. Purusha himself does not execute; he maintains Prakriti in her action and allows her to express in energy and process and formed result what he perceives in his knowledge. This is the distinction made by the Sankhyas; and although it is not all the true truth, not in any way the highest truth either of Purusha or of Prakriti, still it is a valid and indispensable practical knowledge in the lower hemisphere of existence.

The individual soul or the conscious being in a form may identify itself with this experiencing Purusha or with this active Prakriti. If it identifies itself with Prakriti, it is not master, enjoyer and knower, but reflects the modes and workings of Prakriti. It enters by its identification into that subjection and mechanical working which is characteristic of her. And even, by an entire immersion in Prakriti, this soul becomes inconscient or subconscient, asleep in her forms as in the earth and the metal or almost asleep as in plant life. There, in that inconscience, it is subject to the domination of tamas, the principle, the power, the qualitative mode of obscurity and inertia: sattwa and rajas are there, but they are concealed in the thick coating of tamas. Emerging into its own proper nature of consciousness but not yet truly conscious, because there is still too great a domination of tamas in the nature, the embodied being becomes more and more subject to rajas, the principle, the power, the qualitative mode of action and passion impelled by desire and instinct. There is then formed and developed the animal nature, narrow in consciousness, rudimentary in intelligence, rajaso-tamasic in vital habit and impulse. Emerging yet farther from the great Inconscience towards a spiritual status the embodied being liberates sattwa, the mode of light, and acquires a relative freedom and mastery and knowledge and with it a qualified and conditioned sense of inner satisfaction and happiness. Man, the mental being in a physical body, should be but is not, except in a few among this multitude of ensouled bodies, of this nature. Ordinarily he has too much in him of the obscure earth-inertia and a troubled ignorant animal life-force to be a soul of light and bliss or even a mind of harmonious will and knowledge. There is here in man an incomplete and still hampered and baffled ascension towards the true character of the Purusha, free, master, knower and enjoyer. For these are in human and earthly experience relative modes, none giving its single and absolute fruit; all are intermixed with each other and there is not the pure action of any one of them anywhere. It is their confused and inconstant interaction that determines the experiences of the egoistic human consciousness swinging in Nature's uncertain balance.

The sign of the immersion of the embodied soul in Prakriti is the limitation of consciousness to the ego. The vivid stamp of this limited consciousness can be seen in a constant inequality of the mind and heart and a confused conflict and disharmony in their varied reactions to the touches of experience. The human reactions sway perpetually between the dualities created by the soul's subjection to Nature and by its often intense but narrow struggle for mastery and enjoyment, a struggle for the most part ineffective. The soul circles in an unending round of Nature's alluring and distressing opposites, success and failure, good fortune and ill fortune, good and evil, sin and virtue, joy and grief, pain and pleasure. It is only when, awaking from its immersion in Prakriti, it perceives its oneness with the One and its oneness with all existences that it can become free from these things and found its right relation to this executive world-Nature. Then it becomes indifferent to her inferior modes, equal-minded to her dualities, capable of mastery and freedom; it is seated above her as the high-throned knower and witness filled with the calm intense unalloyed delight of his own eternal existence. The embodied spirit continues to express its powers in action, but it is no longer involved in ignorance, no longer bound by its works; its actions have no longer a consequence within it, but only a consequence outside in Prakriti. The whole movement of Nature becomes to its experience a rising and falling of waves on the surface that make no difference to its own unfathomable peace, its wide delight, its vast universal equality or its boundless God-existence.[3]

~

These are the conditions of our effort and they point to an ideal which can be expressed in these or in equivalent formulae.

To live in God and not in the ego; to move, vastly founded, not in the little egoistic consciousness, but in the consciousness of the All-Soul and the Transcendent.

To be perfectly equal in all happenings and to all beings, and to see and feel them as one with oneself and one with the Divine; to feel all in oneself and all in God; to feel God in all, oneself in all.

To act in God and not in the ego. And here, first, not to choose action by reference to personal needs and standards, but in obedience to the dictates of the living highest Truth above us. Next, as soon as we are sufficiently founded in the spiritual consciousness, not to act any longer by our separate will or movement, but more and more to allow action to happen and develop under the impulsion and guidance of a divine Will that surpasses us. And last, the supreme result, to be exalted into an identity in knowledge, force, consciousness, act, joy of existence with the Divine Shakti; to feel a dynamic movement not dominated by mortal desire and vital instinct and impulse and illusive mental free-will, but luminously conceived and evolved in an immortal self-delight and an infinite self-knowledge. For this is the action that comes by a conscious subjection and merging of the natural man into the divine Self and eternal Spirit; it is the Spirit that for ever transcends and guides this world-Nature.

But by what practical steps of self-discipline can we arrive at this consummation?

The elimination of all egoistic activity and of its foundation, the egoistic consciousness, is clearly the key to the consummation we desire. And since in the path of works action is the knot we have first to loosen, we must endeavour to loosen it where it is centrally tied, in desire and in ego; for otherwise we shall cut only stray strands and not the heart of our bondage. These are the two knots of our subjection to this ignorant and divided Nature, desire and ego-sense. And of these two desire has its native home in the emotions and sensations and instincts and from there affects thought and volition; ego-sense lives indeed in these movements, but it casts its deep roots also in the thinking mind and its will and it is there that it becomes fully self-conscious. These are the twin obscure powers of the obsessing world-wide Ignorance that we have to enlighten and eliminate.

In the field of action desire takes many forms, but the most powerful of all is the vital self's craving or seeking after the fruit of our works. The fruit we covet may be a reward of internal pleasure; it may be the accomplishment of some preferred idea or some cherished will or the satisfaction of the egoistic emotions, or else the pride of success of our highest hopes and ambitions. Or it may be an external reward, a recompense entirely material,—wealth, position, honour, victory, good fortune or any other fulfilment of vital or physical desire. But all alike are lures by which egoism holds us. Always these satisfactions delude us with the sense of mastery and the idea of freedom, while really we are harnessed and guided or ridden and whipped by some gross or subtle, some noble or ignoble, figure of the blind Desire that drives the world. Therefore the first rule of action laid down by the Gita is to do the work that should be done without any desire for the fruit, *niṣkāma karma*.

A simple rule in appearance, and yet how difficult to carry out with anything like an absolute sincerity and liberating entireness! In the greater part of our action we use the principle very little if at all, and then even mostly as a sort of counterpoise to the normal principle of desire and to mitigate the extreme action of that tyrant impulse. At best, we are satisfied if we arrive at a modified and disciplined egoism not too shocking to our moral sense, not too brutally offensive to others. And to our partial self-discipline we give various names and forms; we habituate ourselves by practice to the sense of duty, to a firm fidelity to principle, a stoical fortitude or a religious resignation, a quiet or an ecstatic submission to God's will. But it is not these things that the Gita intends, useful though they are in their place; it aims at something absolute, unmitigated, uncompromising, a turn, an attitude that will change the whole poise of the soul. Not the mind's control of vital impulse is its rule, but the strong immobility of an immortal spirit.

The test it lays down is an absolute equality of the mind and the heart to all results, to all reactions, to all happenings. If good fortune and ill fortune, if respect and insult, if reputation and obloquy, if victory and defeat, if pleasant event and sorrowful event leave us not only unshaken but untouched, free in the emotions, free in the nervous reactions, free in the mental view, not responding with the least disturbance or vibration in any spot of the nature, then we have the absolute liberation to which the Gita points us, but not otherwise. The tiniest reaction is a proof that the discipline is imperfect and that some part of us accepts ignorance and bondage as its law and clings still to the old nature. Our self-conquest is only partially accomplished; it is still imperfect or unreal in some stretch or part or smallest spot of the ground of our nature. And that little pebble of imperfection may throw down the whole achievement of the Yoga!

There are certain semblances of an equal spirit which must not be mistaken for the profound and vast spiritual equality which the Gita teaches. There is an equality of disappointed resignation, an equality of pride, an equality of hardness and indifference: all these are egoistic in their nature. Inevitably they come in the course of the sadhana, but they must be rejected or transformed into the true quietude. There is too, on a higher level, the equality of the stoic, the equality of a devout resignation or a sage detachment, the equality of a soul aloof from the world and indifferent to its doings. These too are insufficient; first approaches they can be, but they are at most early soul-phases only or imperfect mental preparations for our entry into the true and absolute self-existent wide evenness of the spirit.

For it is certain that so great a result cannot be arrived at immediately and without any previous stages. At first we have to learn to bear the shocks of the world with the central part of our being untouched and silent, even when the surface mind, heart, life are strongly shaken; unmoved there on the bedrock of our life, we must separate the soul watching behind or immune deep within from these outer workings of our nature. Afterwards, extending this calm and steadfastness of the detached soul to its instruments, it will become slowly possible to radiate peace from the luminous centre to the darker peripheries. In this process we may take the passing help of many minor phases; a certain stoicism, a certain calm philosophy, a certain religious exaltation may help us towards some nearness to our aim, or we may call in even less strong and exalted but still useful powers of our mental nature. In the end we must either discard or transform them and arrive instead at an entire equality, a perfect self-existent peace within and even, if we can, a total unassailable, self-poised and spontaneous delight in all our members.

But how then shall we continue to act at all? For ordinarily the human being acts because he has a desire or feels a mental, vital or physical want or need; he is driven by the necessities of the body, by the lust of riches, honours or fame, or by a craving for the personal satisfactions of the mind or the heart or a craving for power or pleasure. Or he is seized and pushed about by a moral need or, at least, the need or the desire of making his ideas or his ideals or his will or his party or his country or his gods prevail in the world. If none of these desires nor any other must be the spring of our action, it would seem as if all incentive or motive power had been removed and action itself must necessarily cease. The Gita replies with its third great secret of the divine life. All action must be done in a more and more Godward and finally a God-possessed consciousness; our works must be a sacrifice to the Divine and in the end a surrender of all our being, mind, will, heart, sense, life and body to the One must make God-love and God-service our only motive. This transformation of the motive force and very character of works is indeed its master idea; it is the foundation of its unique synthesis of works, love and knowledge. In the end not desire, but the consciously felt will of the Eternal remains as the sole driver of our action and the sole originator of its initiative.

Equality, renunciation of all desire for the fruit of our works, action done as a sacrifice to the supreme Lord of our nature and of all nature,—these are the three first Godward approaches in the Gita's way of Karmayoga.

---

1. *rahasyam uttamam.*
2. This Power is the conscious divine Shakti of the Ishwara, the transcendent and universal Mother.

3. It is not indispensable for the Karmayoga to accept implicitly all the philosophy of the Gita. We may regard it, if we like, as a statement of psychological experience useful as a practical basis for the Yoga; here it is perfectly valid and in entire consonance with a high and wide experience. For this reason I have thought it well to state it here, as far as possible in the language of modern thought, omitting all that belongs to metaphysics rather than to psychology.

CHAPTER IV. THE SACRIFICE, THE TRIUNE PATH AND THE LORD OF THE SACRIFICE

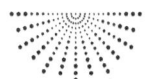

THE LAW of sacrifice is the common divine action that was thrown out into the world in its beginning as a symbol of the solidarity of the universe. It is by the attraction of this law that a divinising principle, a saving power descends to limit and correct and gradually to eliminate the errors of an egoistic and self-divided creation. This descent, this sacrifice of the Purusha, the Divine Soul submitting itself to Force and Matter so that it may inform and illuminate them, is the seed of redemption of this world of Inconscience and Ignorance. "For with sacrifice as their companion," says the Gita, "the All-Father created these peoples." The acceptance of the law of sacrifice is a practical recognition by the ego that it is neither alone in the world nor chief in the world. It is its admission that, even in this much fragmented existence, there is beyond itself and behind that which is not its own egoistic person, something greater and completer, a diviner All which demands from it subordination and service. Indeed, sacrifice is imposed and, where need be, compelled by the universal World-Force; it takes it even from those who do not consciously recognise the law,—inevitably, because this is the intrinsic nature of things. Our ignorance or our false egoistic view of life can make no difference to this eternal bedrock truth of Nature. For this is the truth in Nature, that this ego which thinks itself a separate independent being and claims to live for itself, is not and cannot be independent nor separate, nor can it live to itself even if it would, but rather all are linked together by a secret Oneness. Each existence is continually giving out perforce from its stock; out of its mental receipts from Nature or its vital and physical assets and acquisitions and belongings a stream goes to all that is around it. And always again it receives something from its environment gratis or in return for its voluntary or involuntary tribute. For it is only by this giving and receiving that it can effect its own growth while at the same time it helps the sum of things. At length, though at first slowly and partially, we learn to make the conscious sacrifice; even, in the end, we take joy to give ourselves and what we envisage as belonging to us in a spirit of love and devotion to That which appears for the moment other than ourselves and is certainly other than our limited personalities. The sacrifice and the divine return for our sacrifice then become a gladly accepted means towards our last perfection; for it is recognised now as the road to the fulfilment in us of the eternal purpose.

But, most often, the sacrifice is done unconsciously, egoistically and without knowledge or acceptance of the true meaning of the great world-rite. It is so that the vast majority of earth-creatures do it; and, when it is so done, the individual derives only a mechanical minimum of natural inevitable profit, achieves by it only a slow painful progress limited and tortured by the smallness and suffering of the ego. Only when the heart, the will and the mind of knowledge associate themselves with the law and gladly follow it, can there come the deep joy and the happy fruitfulness of divine sacrifice. The mind's knowledge of the law and the heart's gladness in it culminate in the perception that it is to our own Self and Spirit and the one Self and Spirit of all that we give. And this is true even when our self-offering is still to our fellow-creatures or to lesser Powers and Principles and not yet to the Supreme. "Not for the sake of the wife," says Yajnavalkya in the Upanishad, "but for the sake of the Self is the wife dear to us." This in the lower sense of the individual self is the hard fact behind the coloured and passionate professions of egoistic love; but in a higher sense it is the inner significance of that love too which is not egoistic but divine. All true love and all sacrifice are in their essence Nature's contradiction of the primary egoism and its separative error; it is her attempt to turn from a necessary first fragmentation towards a recovered oneness. All unity between creatures is in its essence a self-finding, a fusion with that from which we have separated, a discovery of one's self in others.

But it is only a divine love and unity that can possess in the light what the human forms of these things seek for in the darkness. For the true unity is not merely an association and agglomeration like that of physical cells joined by a life of common interests; it is not even an emotional understanding, sympathy, solidarity or close drawing together. Only then are we really unified with those separated from us by the divisions of Nature, when we annul the division and find ourselves in that which seemed to us not ourselves. Association is a vital and physical unity; its sacrifice is that of mutual aid and concessions. Nearness, sympathy, solidarity create a mental, moral and emotional unity; theirs is a sacrifice of mutual support and mutual gratifications. But the true unity is spiritual; its sacrifice is a mutual self-giving, an interfusion of our inner substance.

The law of sacrifice travels in Nature towards its culmination in this complete and unreserved self-giving; it awakens the consciousness of one common self in the giver and the object of the sacrifice. This culmination of sacrifice is the height even of human love and devotion when it tries to become divine; for there too the highest peak of love points into a heaven of complete mutual self-giving, its summit is the rapturous fusing of two souls into one.

This profounder idea of the world-wide law is at the heart of the teaching about works given in the Gita; a spiritual union with the Highest by sacrifice, an unreserved self-giving to the Eternal is the core of its doctrine. The vulgar conception of sacrifice is an act of painful self-immolation, austere self-mortification, difficult self-effacement; this kind of sacrifice may go even as far as self-mutilation and self-torture. These things may be temporarily necessary in man's hard endeavour to exceed his natural self; if the egoism in his nature is violent and obstinate, it has to be met sometimes by an answering strong internal repression and counterbalancing violence. But the Gita discourages any excess of violence done to oneself; for the self within is really the Godhead evolving, it is Krishna, it is the Divine; it has not to be troubled and tortured as the Titans of the world trouble and torture it, but to be increased, fostered, cherished, luminously opened to a divine light and strength and joy and wideness. It is not one's self, but the band of the spirit's inner enemies that we have to discourage, expel, slay upon the altar of the growth of the spirit; these can be ruthlessly excised, whose names are desire, wrath, inequality, greed, attachment to outward pleasures and pains, the cohort of usurping demons that are the cause of the soul's errors and sufferings. These should be regarded not as part of oneself but as intruders and perverters of our self's real and diviner nature; these have to be sacrificed in the harsher sense of the word, whatever pain in going they may throw by reflection on the consciousness of the seeker.

But the true essence of sacrifice is not self-immolation, it is self-giving; its object not self-effacement, but self-fulfilment; its method not self-mortification, but a greater life, not self-mutilation, but a transformation of our natural human parts into divine members, not self-torture, but a passage from a lesser satisfaction to a greater Ananda. There is only one thing painful in the beginning to a raw or turbid part of the surface nature; it is the indispensable discipline demanded, the denial necessary for the merging of the incomplete ego. But for that there can be a speedy and enormous compensation in the discovery of a real greater or ultimate completeness in others, in all things, in the cosmic oneness, in the freedom of the transcendent Self and Spirit, in the rapture of the touch of the Divine. Our sacrifice is not a giving without any return or any fruitful acceptance from the other side; it is an interchange between the embodied soul and conscious Nature in us and the eternal Spirit. For even though no return is demanded, yet there is the knowledge deep within us that a marvellous return is inevitable. The soul knows that it does not give itself to God in vain; claiming nothing, it yet receives the infinite riches of the divine Power and Presence.

Last, there is to be considered the recipient of the sacrifice and the manner of the sacrifice. The sacrifice may be offered to others or it may be offered to divine Powers; it may be offered to the cosmic All or it may be offered to the transcendent Supreme. The worship given may take any shape from the dedication of a leaf or flower, a cup of water, a handful of rice, a loaf of bread, to consecration of all that we possess and the submission of all that we are. Whoever the recipient, whatever the gift, it is the Supreme, the Eternal in things, who receives and accepts it, even if it be rejected or ignored by the immediate recipient. For the Supreme who transcends the universe, is yet here too, however veiled, in us and in the world and in its happenings; he is there as the omniscient Witness and Receiver of all our works and their secret Master. All our actions, all our efforts, even our sins and stumblings and sufferings and struggles are obscurely or consciously, known to us and seen or else unknown and in a disguise, governed in their last result by the One. All is turned towards him in his numberless forms and offered through them to the single Omnipresence. In whatever form and with whatever spirit we approach him, in that form and with that spirit he receives the sacrifice.

And the fruit also of the sacrifice of works varies according to the work, according to the intention in the work and according to the spirit that is behind the intention. But all other sacrifices are partial, egoistic, mixed, temporal, incomplete,—even those offered to the highest Powers and Principles keep this character: the result too is partial, limited, temporal, mixed in its reactions, effective only for a minor or intermediate purpose. The one entirely acceptable sacrifice is a last and highest and uttermost self-giving, —it is that surrender made face to face, with devotion and knowledge, freely and without any reserve to One who is at once our immanent Self, the environing constituent All, the Supreme Reality beyond this or any manifestation and, secretly, all these together, concealed everywhere, the immanent Transcendence. For to the soul that wholly gives itself to him, God also gives himself altogether. Only the one who offers his whole nature, finds the Self. Only the one who can give everything, enjoys the Divine All everywhere. Only a supreme self-abandonment attains to the Supreme. Only the sublimation by sacrifice of all that we are, can enable us to embody the Highest and live here in the immanent consciousness of the transcendent Spirit.

∽

This, in short, is the demand made on us, that we should turn our whole life into a conscious sacrifice. Every moment and every movement of our being is to be resolved into a continuous and a devoted self-giving to the Eternal. All our actions, not less the smallest and most ordinary and trifling than the greatest and most uncommon and noble, must be performed as consecrated acts. Our individualised nature must live in the single consciousness of an inner and outer movement dedicated to Something that is beyond us and greater than our ego. No matter what the gift or to whom it is presented by us, there must be a consciousness in the act that we are presenting it to the one divine Being in all beings. Our commonest or most grossly material actions must assume this sublimated character; when we eat, we should be conscious that we are giving our food to that Presence in us; it must be a sacred offering in a temple and the sense of a mere physical need or self-gratification must pass away from us. In any great labour, in any high discipline, in any difficult or noble enterprise, whether undertaken for ourselves, for others or for the race, it will no longer be possible to stop short at the idea of the race, of ourselves or of others. The thing we are doing must be consciously offered as a sacrifice of works, not to these, but either through them or directly to the One Godhead; the Divine Inhabitant who was hidden by these figures must be no longer hidden but ever present to our soul, our mind, our sense. The workings and results of our acts must be put in the hands of that One in the feeling that that Presence is the Infinite and Most High by whom alone our labour and our aspiration are possible. For in his being all takes place; for him all labour and aspiration are taken from us by Nature and offered on his altar. Even in those things in which Nature is herself very plainly the worker and we only the witnesses of her working and its containers and supporters, there should be the same constant memory and insistent consciousness of a work and of its divine Master. Our very inspiration and respiration, our very heart-beats can and must be made conscious in us as the living rhythm of the universal sacrifice.

It is clear that a conception of this kind and its effective practice must carry in them three results that are of a central importance for our spiritual ideal. It is evident, to begin with, that, even if such a discipline is begun without devotion, it leads straight and inevitably towards the highest devotion possible; for it must deepen naturally into the completest adoration imaginable, the most profound God-love. There is bound up with it a growing sense of the Divine in all things, a deepening communion with the Divine in all our thought, will and action and at every moment of our lives, a more and more moved consecration to the Divine of the totality of our being. Now these implications of the Yoga of works are also of the very essence of an integral and absolute Bhakti. The seeker who puts them into living practice makes in himself continually a constant, active and effective representation of the very spirit of self-devotion, and it is inevitable that out of it there should emerge the most engrossing worship of the Highest to whom is given this service. An absorbing love for the Divine Presence to whom he feels an always more intimate closeness, grows upon the consecrated worker. And with it is born or in it is contained a universal love too for all these beings, living forms and creatures that are habitations of the Divine—not the brief restless grasping emotions of division, but the settled selfless love that is the deeper vibration of oneness. In all the seeker begins to meet the one Object of his adoration and service. The way of works turns by this road of sacrifice to meet the path of Devotion; it can be itself a devotion as complete, as absorbing, as integral as any the desire of the heart can ask for or the passion of the mind can imagine.

Next, the practice of this Yoga demands a constant inward remembrance of the one central liberating knowledge, and a constant active externalising of it in works comes in too to intensify the remembrance. In all is the one Self, the one Divine is all; all are in the Divine, all are the Divine and there is nothing else in the universe,—this thought or this faith is the whole background until it becomes the whole substance of the consciousness of the worker. A memory, a self-dynamising meditation of this kind, must and does in its end turn into a profound and uninterrupted vision and a vivid and all-embracing consciousness of that which we so powerfully remember or on which we so constantly meditate. For it compels a constant reference at each moment to the Origin of all being and will and action and there is at once an embracing and exceeding of all particular forms and appearances in That which is their cause and upholder. This way cannot go to its end without a seeing vivid and vital, as concrete in its way as physical sight, of the works of the universal Spirit everywhere. On its summits it rises into a constant living and thinking and willing and acting in the presence of the Supramental, the Transcendent. Whatever we see and hear, whatever we touch and sense, all of which we are conscious, has to be known and felt by us as That which we worship and serve; all has to be turned into an image of the Divinity, perceived as a dwelling-place of his Godhead, enveloped with the eternal Omnipresence. In its close, if not long before it, this way of works turns by communion with the Divine Presence, Will and Force into a way of Knowledge more complete and integral than any the mere creature intelligence can construct or the search of the intellect can discover.

Lastly, the practice of this Yoga of sacrifice compels us to renounce all the inner supports of egoism, casting them out of our mind and will and actions, and to eliminate its seed, its presence, its influence out of our nature. All must be done for the Divine; all must be directed towards the Divine. Nothing must be attempted for ourselves as a separate existence; nothing done for others, whether neighbours, friends, family, country or mankind or other creatures merely because they are connected with our personal life and thought and sentiment or because the ego takes a preferential interest in their welfare. In this way of doing and seeing all works and all life become only a daily dynamic worship and service of the Divine in the unbounded temple of his own vast cosmic existence. Life becomes more and more the sacrifice of the eternal in the individual constantly self-offered to the eternal Transcendence. It is offered in the wide sacrificial ground of the field of the eternal cosmic Spirit; and the Force too that offers it is the eternal Force, the omnipresent Mother. Therefore is this way a way of union and communion by acts and by the spirit and knowledge in the act as complete and integral as any our Godward will can hope for or our soul's strength execute.

It has all the power of a way of works integral and absolute, but because of its law of sacrifice and self-giving to the Divine Self and Master, it is accompanied on its one side by the whole power of the path of Love and on the other by the whole power of the path of Knowledge. At its end all these three divine Powers work together, fused, united, completed, perfected by each other.

~

The Divine, the Eternal is the Lord of our sacrifice of works and union with him in all our being and consciousness and in its expressive instruments is the one object of the sacrifice; the steps of the sacrifice of works must therefore be measured, first, by the growth in our nature of something that brings us nearer to divine Nature, but secondly also by an experience of the Divine, his presence, his manifestation to us, an increasing closeness and union with that Presence. But the Divine is in his essence infinite and his manifestation too is multitudinously infinite. If that is so, it is not likely that our true integral perfection in being and in nature can come by one kind of realisation alone; it must combine many different strands of divine experience. It cannot be reached by the exclusive pursuit of a single line of identity till that is raised to its absolute; it must harmonise many aspects of the Infinite. An integral consciousness with a multiform dynamic experience is essential for the complete transformation of our nature.

There is one fundamental perception indispensable towards any integral knowledge or many-sided experience of this Infinite. It is to realise the Divine in its essential self and truth unaltered by forms and phenomena. Otherwise we are likely to remain caught in the net of appearances or wander confusedly in a chaotic multitude of cosmic or particular aspects, and if we avoid this confusion, it will be at the price of getting chained to some mental formula or shut up in a limited personal experience. The one secure and all-reconciling truth which is the very foundation of the universe is this that life is the manifestation of an uncreated Self and Spirit, and the key to life's hidden secret is the true relation of this Spirit with its own created existences. There is behind all this life the look of an eternal Being upon its multitudinous becomings; there is around and everywhere in it the envelopment and penetration of a manifestation in time by an unmanifested timeless Eternal. But this knowledge is valueless for Yoga if it is only an intellectual and metaphysical notion void of life and barren of consequence; a mental realisation alone cannot be sufficient for the seeker. For what Yoga searches after is not truth of thought alone or truth of mind alone, but the dynamic truth of a living and revealing spiritual experience. There must awake in us a constant indwelling and enveloping nearness, a vivid perception, a close feeling and communion, a concrete sense and contact of a true and infinite Presence always and everywhere. That Presence must remain with us as the living, pervading Reality in which we and all things exist and move and act, and we must feel it always and everywhere, concrete, visible, inhabiting all things; it must be patent to us as their true Self, tangible as their imperishable Essence, met by us closely as their inmost Spirit. To see, to feel, to sense, to contact in every way and not merely to conceive this Self and Spirit here in all existences and to feel with the same vividness all existences in this Self and Spirit, is the fundamental experience which must englobe all other knowledge.

This infinite and eternal Self of things is an omnipresent Reality, one existence everywhere; it is a single unifying presence and not different in different creatures; it can be met, seen or felt in its completeness in each soul or each form in the universe. For its infinity is spiritual and essential and not merely a boundlessness in Space or an endlessness in Time; the Infinite can be felt in an infinitesimal atom or in a second of time as convincingly as in the stretch of the aeons or the stupendous enormity of the intersolar spaces. The knowledge or experience of it can begin anywhere and express itself through anything; for the Divine is in all, and all is the Divine.

This fundamental experience will yet begin differently for different natures and take long to develop all the Truth that it conceals in its thousand aspects. I see perhaps or feel in myself or as myself first the eternal Presence and afterwards only can extend the vision or sense of this greater self of mine to all creatures. I then see the world in me or as one with me. I perceive the universe as a scene in my being, the play of its processes as a movement of forms and souls and forces in my cosmic spirit; I meet myself and none else everywhere. Not, be it well noted, with the error of the Asura, the Titan, who lives in his own inordinately magnified shadow, mistakes ego for the self and spirit and tries to impose his fragmentary personality as the one dominant existence upon all his surroundings. For, having the knowledge, I have already seized this reality that my true self is the non-ego, so always my greater Self is felt by me either as an impersonal vastness or an essential Person containing yet beyond all personalities or as both these together; but in any case, whether Impersonal or illimitable Personal or both together, it is an ego-exceeding Infinite. If I have sought it out and found it first in the form of it I call myself rather than in others, it is only because there it is easiest for me, owing to the subjectivity of my consciousness, to find it, to know it at once and to realise it. But if the narrow instrumental ego does not begin to merge in this Self as soon as it is seen, if the smaller external mindconstructed I refuses to disappear into that greater permanent uncreated spiritual I, then my realisation is either not genuine or radically imperfect. There is somewhere in me an egoistic obstacle; some part of my nature has opposed a self-regarding and self-preserving denial to the all-swallowing truth of the Spirit.

On the other hand—and to some this is an easier way—I may see the Divinity first in the world outside me, not in myself but in others. I meet it there from the beginning as an indwelling and all-containing Infinite that is not bound up with all these forms, creatures and forces which it bears on its surface. Or else I see and feel it as a pure solitary Self and Spirit which contains all these powers and existences, and I lose my sense of ego in the silent Omnipresence around me. Afterwards it is this that begins to pervade and possess my instrumental being and out of it seem to proceed all my impulsions to action, all my light of thought and speech, all the formations of my consciousness and all its relations and impacts with other soul-forms of this one worldwide Existence. I am already no longer this little personal self, but That with something of itself put forward which sustains a selected form of its workings in the universe.

There is another basic realisation, the most extreme of all, that yet comes sometimes as the first decisive opening or an early turn of the Yoga. It is the awakening to an ineffable high transcendent Unknowable above myself and above this world in which I seem to move, a timeless and spaceless condition or entity which is at once, in some way compelling and convincing to an essential consciousness in me, the one thing that is to it overwhelmingly real. This experience is usually accompanied by an equally compelling sense either of the dreamlike or shadowy illusoriness of all things here or else of their temporary, derivative and only half-real character. For a time at least all around me may seem to be a moving of cinematographic shadow forms or surface figures and my own action may appear as a fluid formulation from some Source ungrasped as yet and perhaps unseizable above or outside me. To remain in this consciousness, to carry out this initiation or follow out this first suggestion of the character of things would be to proceed towards the goal of dissolution of self and world in the Unknowable,—Moksha, Nirvana. But this is not the only line of issue; it is possible, on the contrary, for me to wait till through the silence of this timeless unfilled liberation I begin to enter into relations with that yet ungrasped Source of myself and my actions; then the void begins to fill, there emerges out of it or there rushes into it all the manifold Truth of the Divine, all the aspects and manifestations and many levels of a dynamic Infinite. At first this experience imposes on the mind and then on all our being an absolute, a fathomless, almost an abysmal peace and silence. Overpowered and subjugated, stilled, liberated from itself, the mind accepts the Silence itself as the Supreme. But afterwards the seeker discovers that all is there for him contained or new-made in that silence or through it descends upon him from a greater concealed transcendent Existence. For this Transcendent, this Absolute is not a mere peace of signless emptiness; it has its own infinite contents and riches of which ours are debased and diminished values. If there were not that Source of all things, there could be no universe; all powers, all works and activities would be an illusion, all creation and manifestation would be impossible.

These are the three fundamental realisations, so fundamental that to the Yogin of the way of Knowledge they seem ultimate, sufficient in themselves, destined to overtop and replace all others. And yet for the integral seeker, whether accorded to him at an early stage suddenly and easily by a miraculous grace or achieved with difficulty after a long progress and endeavour, they are neither the sole truth nor the full and only clues to the integral truth of the Eternal, but rather the unfilled beginning, the vast foundation of a greater divine Knowledge. Other realisations there are that are imperatively needed and must be explored to the full limit of their possibilities; and if some of them appear to a first sight to cover only Divine Aspects that are instrumental to the activity of existence but not inherent in its essence, yet, when followed to their end through that activity to its everlasting Source, it is found that they lead to a disclosure of the Divine without which our knowledge of the Truth behind things would be left bare and incomplete. These seeming Instrumentals are the key to a secret without which the Fundamentals themselves would not unveil all their mystery. All the revelatory aspect of the Divine must be caught in the wide net of the integral Yoga.

If a departure from the world and its activities, a supreme release and quietude were the sole aim of the seeker, the three great fundamental realisations would be sufficient for the fulfilment of his spiritual life: concentrated in them alone he could suffer all other divine or mundane knowledge to fall away from him and himself unencumbered, depart into the eternal Silence. But he has to take account of the world and its activities, learn what divine truth there may be behind them and reconcile that apparent opposition between the Divine Truth and the manifest creation which is the starting-point of most spiritual experience. Here, on each line of approach that he can take, he is confronted with a constant Duality, a separation between two terms of existence that seem to be opposites and their opposition to be the very root of the riddle of the universe. Later, he may and does discover that these are the two poles of One Being, connected by two simultaneous currents of energy negative and positive in relation to each other, their interaction the very condition for the manifestation of what is within the Being, their reunion the appointed means for the reconciliation of life's discords and for the discovery of the integral truth of which he is the seeker.

For on one side he is aware of this Self everywhere, this everlasting Spirit-Substance—Brahman, the Eternal—the same self-existence here in time behind each appearance he sees or senses and timeless beyond the universe. He has this strong overpowering experience of a Self that is neither our limited ego nor our mind, life or body, world-wide but not outwardly phenomenal, yet to some spirit-sense in him more concrete than any form or phenomenon, universal yet not dependent for its being on anything in the universe or on the whole totality of the universe; if all this were to disappear, its extinction would make no difference to this Eternal of his constant intimate experience. He is sure of an inexpressible Self-Existence which is the essence of himself and all things; he is intimately aware of an essential Consciousness of which thinking mind and life-sense and bodysense are only partial and diminished figures, a Consciousness with an illimitable Force in it of which all energies are the outcome, but which is yet not explained or accounted for by the sum or power or nature of all these energies together; he feels, he lives in an inalienable self-existent Bliss which is not this lesser transient joy or happiness or pleasure. A changeless imperishable infinity, a timeless eternity, a self-awareness which is not this receptive and reactive or tentacular mental consciousness, but is behind and above it and present too below it, even in what we call Inconscience, a oneness in which there is no possibility of any other existence, are the fourfold character of this settled experience. Yet this eternal Self-Existence is seen by him also as a conscious Time-Spirit bearing the stream of happenings, a self-extended spiritual Space containing all things and beings, a Spirit-Substance which is the very form and material of all that seems non-spiritual, temporary and finite. For all that is transitory, temporal, spatial, bounded, is yet felt by him to be in its substance and energy and power no other than the One, the Eternal, the Infinite.

And yet there is not only in him or before him this eternal self-aware Existence, this spiritual Consciousness, this infinity of self-illumined Force, this timeless and endless Beatitude. There is too, constant also to his experience, this universe in measurable Space and Time, some kind perhaps of boundless finite, and in it all is transient, limited, fragmentary, plural, ignorant, exposed to disharmony and suffering, seeking vaguely for some unrealised yet inherent harmony of oneness, unconscious or half-conscious or, even when most conscious, still tied to the original Ignorance and

Inconscience. He is not always in a trance of peace or bliss and, even if he were, it would be no solution, for he knows that this would still be going on outside him and yet within some larger self of him as if for ever. At times these two states of his spirit seem to exist for him alternately according to his state of consciousness; at others they are there as two parts of his being, disparate and to be reconciled, two halves, an upper and a lower or an inner and an outer half of his existence. He finds soon that this separation in his consciousness has an immense liberative power; for by it he is no longer bound to the Ignorance, the Inconscience; it no longer appears to him the very nature of himself and things but an illusion which can be overcome or at least a temporary wrong self-experience, Maya. It is tempting to regard it as only a contradiction of the Divine, an incomprehensible mystery-play, masque or travesty of the Infinite—and so it irresistibly seems to his experience at times, on one side the luminous verity of Brahman, on the other a dark illusion of Maya. But something in him will not allow him to cut existence thus permanently in two and, looking more closely, he discovers that in this half-light or darkness too is the Eternal—it is the Brahman who is here with this face of Maya.

This is the beginning of a growing spiritual experience which reveals to him more and more that what seemed to him dark incomprehensible Maya was all the time no other than the Consciousness-Puissance of the Eternal, timeless and illimitable beyond the universe, but spread out here under a mask of bright and dark opposites for the miracle of the slow manifestation of the Divine in Mind and Life and Matter. All the Timeless presses towards the play in Time; all in Time turns upon and around the timeless Spirit. If the separate experience was liberative, this unitive experience is dynamic and effective. For he now not only feels himself to be in his soul-substance part of the Eternal, in his essential self and spirit entirely one with the Eternal, but in his active nature an instrumentation of its omniscient and omnipotent Consciousness-Puissance. However bounded and relative its present play in him, he can open to a greater and greater consciousness and power of it and to that expansion there seems to be no assignable limit. A level spiritual and supramental of that Consciousness-Puissance seems even to reveal itself above him and lean to enter into contact, where there are not these trammels and limits, and its powers too are pressing upon the play in Time with the promise of a greater descent and a less disguised or no longer disguised manifestation of the Eternal. The once conflicting but now biune duality of Brahman-Maya stands revealed to him as the first great dynamic aspect of the Self of all selves, the Master of existence, the Lord of the world-sacrifice and of his sacrifice.

On another line of approach another Duality presents itself to the experience of the seeker. On one side he becomes aware of a witness recipient observing experiencing Consciousness which does not appear to act but for which all these activities inside and outside us seem to be undertaken and continue. On the other side he is aware at the same time of an executive Force or an energy of Process which is seen to constitute, drive and guide all conceivable activities and to create a myriad forms visible to us and invisible and use them as stable supports for its incessant flux of action and creation. Entering exclusively into the witness consciousness he becomes silent, untouched, immobile; he sees that he has till now passively reflected and appropriated to himself the movements of Nature and it is by this reflection that they acquired from the witness soul within him what seemed a spiritual value and significance. But now he has withdrawn that ascription or mirroring identification; he is conscious only of his silent self and aloof from all that is in motion around it; all activities are outside him and at once they cease to be intimately real; they appear now mechanical, detachable, endable. Entering exclusively into the kinetic movement, he has an opposite self-awareness; he seems to his own perception a mass of activities, a formation and result of forces; if there is an active consciousness, even some kind of kinetic being in the midst of it all, yet there is no longer a free soul in it anywhere. These two different and opposite states of being alternate in him or else stand simultaneously over against each other; one silent in the inner being observes but is unmoved and does not participate; the other active in some outer or surface self pursues its habitual movements. He has entered into an intense separative perception of the great duality, Soul-Nature, Purusha-Prakriti.

But as the consciousness deepens, he becomes aware that this is only a first frontal appearance. For he finds that it is by the silent support, permission or sanction of this witness soul in him that this executive nature can work intimately or persistently upon his being; if the soul withdraws its sanction, the movements of Nature in their action upon and within him become a wholly mechanical repetition, vehement at first as if seeking still to enforce their hold, but afterwards less and less dynamic and real. More actively using this power of sanction or refusal, he perceives that he can, slowly and uncertainly at first, more decisively afterwards, change the movements of Nature. Eventually in this witness soul or behind it is revealed to him the presence of a Knower and master Will in Nature, and all her activities more and more appear as an expression of what is known and either actively willed or passively permitted by this Lord of her existence. Prakriti herself now seems to be mechanical only in the carefully regulated appearance of her workings, but in fact a conscious Force with a soul within her, a self-aware significance in her turns, a revelation of a secret Will and Knowledge in her steps and figures. This Duality, in aspect separate, is inseparable. Wherever there is Prakriti, there is Purusha; wherever there is Purusha, there is Prakriti. Even in his inactivity he holds in himself all her force and energies ready for projection; even in the drive of her action she carries with her all his observing and mandatory consciousness as the whole support and sense of her creative purpose. Once more the seeker discovers in his experience the two poles of existence of One Being and the two lines or currents of their energy negative and positive in relation to each other which effect by their simultaneity the manifestation of all that is within it. Here too he finds that the separative aspect is liberative; for it releases him from the bondage of identification with the inadequate workings of Nature in the Ignorance. The unitive aspect is dynamic and effective; for it enables him to arrive at mastery and perfection; while rejecting what is less divine or seemingly undivine in her, he can rebuild her forms and movements in himself according to a nobler pattern and the law and rhythm of a greater existence. At a certain spiritual and supramental level the Duality becomes still more perfectly Two-in-one, the Master Soul with the Conscious Force within it, and its potentiality disowns all barriers and breaks through every limit. Thus this once separate, now biune Duality of Purusha-Prakriti is revealed to him in all its truth as the second great instrumental and effective aspect of the Soul of all souls, the Master of existence, the Lord of the Sacrifice.

On yet another line of approach the seeker meets another corresponding but in aspect distinct Duality in which the biune character is more immediately apparent,—the dynamic Duality of Ishwara-Shakti. On one side he is aware of an infinite and self-existent Godhead in being who contains all things in an ineffable potentiality of existence, a Self of all selves, a Soul of all souls, a spiritual Substance of all substances, an impersonal inexpressible Existence, but at the same time an illimitable Person who is here self-represented in numberless personality, a Master of Knowledge, a Master of Forces, a Lord of love and bliss and beauty, a single Origin of the worlds, a self-manifester and self-creator, a Cosmic Spirit, a universal Mind, a universal Life, the conscious and living Reality supporting the appearance which we sense as unconscious inanimate Matter. On the other side he becomes aware of the same Godhead in effectuating consciousness and power put forth as a self-aware Force that contains and carries all within her and is charged to manifest it in universal Time and Space. It is evident to him that here there is one supreme and infinite Being represented to us in two different sides of itself, obverse and reverse in relation to each other. All is either prepared or pre-existent in the Godhead in Being and issues from it and is upheld by its Will and Presence; all is brought out, carried in movement by the Godhead in power; all becomes and acts and develops by her and in her its individual or its cosmic purpose. It is again a Duality necessary for the manifestation, creating and enabling that double current of energy which seems always necessary for the world-workings, two poles of the same Being, but here closer to each other and always very evidently carrying each the powers of the other in its essence and its dynamic nature. At the same time by the fact that the two great elements of the divine Mystery, the Personal and the Impersonal, are here fused together, the seeker of the integral Truth feels in the duality of Ishwara-Shakti his closeness to a more intimate and ultimate secret of the divine Transcendence and the Manifestation than that offered to him by any other experience.

For the Ishwari Shakti, divine Conscious-Force and WorldMother, becomes a mediatrix between the eternal One and the manifested Many. On one side, by the play of the energies which she brings from the One, she manifests the multiple Divine in the universe, involving and evolving its endless appearances out of her revealing substance; on the other by the reascending current of the same energies she leads back all towards That from which they have issued so that the soul in its evolutionary manifestation may more and more return towards the Divinity there or here put on its divine character. There is not in her, although she devises a cosmic mechanism, the character of an inconscient mechanical Executrix which we find in the first physiognomy of Prakriti, the Nature-Force; neither is there that sense of an Unreality, creatrix of illusions or semi-illusions, which is attached to our first view of Maya. It is at once clear to the experiencing soul that here is a conscious Power of one substance and nature with the Supreme from whom she came. If she seems to have plunged us into the Ignorance and Inconscience in pursuance of a plan we cannot yet interpret, if her forces present themselves as all these ambiguous forces of the universe, yet it becomes visible before long that she is working for the development of the Divine Consciousness in us and that she stands above drawing us to her own higher entity, revealing to us more and more the very essence of the Divine Knowledge, Will and Ananda. Even in the movements of the Ignorance the soul of the seeker becomes aware of her conscious guidance supporting his steps and leading them slowly or swiftly, straight or by many detours out of the darkness into the light of a greater consciousness, out of mortality into immortality, out of evil and suffering towards a highest good and felicity of which as yet his human mind can form only a faint image. Thus her power is at once liberative and dynamic, creative, effective,—creative not only of things as they are, but of things that are to be; for, eliminating the twisted and tangled movements of his lower consciousness made of the stuff of the Ignorance, it rebuilds and new-makes his soul and nature into the substance and forces of a higher divine Nature.

In this Duality too there is possible a separative experience. At one pole of it the seeker may be conscious only of the Master of Existence putting forth on him His energies of knowledge, power and bliss to liberate and divinise; the Shakti may appear to him only an impersonal Force expressive of these things or an attribute of the Ishwara. At the other pole he may encounter the World-Mother, creatrix of the universe, putting forth the Gods and the worlds and all things and existences out of her spirit-substance. Or even if he sees both aspects, it may be with an unequal separating vision, subordinating one to the other, regarding the Shakti only as a means for approaching the Ishwara. There results a one-sided tendency or a lack of balance, a power of effectuation not perfectly supported or a light of revelation not perfectly dynamic. It is when a complete union of the two sides of the Duality is effected and rules his consciousness that he begins to open to a fuller power that will draw him altogether out of the confused clash of Ideas and Forces here into a higher Truth and enable the descent of that Truth to illumine and deliver and act sovereignly upon this world of Ignorance. He has begun to lay his hand on the integral secret which in its fullness can be grasped only when he overpasses the double term that reigns here of Knowledge inextricably intertwined with an original Ignorance and crosses the border where spiritual mind disappears into supramental Gnosis. It is through this third and most dynamic dual aspect of the One that the seeker begins with the most integral completeness to enter into the deepest secret of the being of the Lord of the Sacrifice.

For it is behind the mystery of the presence of personality in an apparently impersonal universe—as in that of consciousness manifesting out of the Inconscient, life out of the inanimate, soul out of brute Matter—that is hidden the solution of the riddle of existence. Here again is another dynamic Duality more pervading than appears at first view and deeply necessary to the play of the slowly self-revealing Power. It is possible for the seeker in his spiritual experience, standing at one pole of the Duality, to follow Mind in seeing a fundamental Impersonality everywhere. The evolving soul in the material world begins from a vast impersonal Inconscience in which our inner sight yet perceives the presence of a veiled infinite Spirit; it proceeds with the emergence of a precarious consciousness and personality that even at their fullest have the look of an episode, but an episode that repeats itself in a constant series; it arises through experience of life out of mind into an infinite, impersonal and absolute Superconscience in which personality, mind-consciousness, life-consciousness seem all to disappear by a liberating annihilation, Nirvana. At a lower pitch he still experiences this fundamental impersonality as an immense liberating force everywhere. It releases his knowledge from the narrowness of personal mind, his will from the clutch of personal desire, his heart from the bondage of petty mutable emotions, his life from its petty personal groove, his soul from ego, and it allows them to embrace calm, equality, wideness, universality, infinity. A Yoga of works would seem to require Personality as its mainstay, almost its source, but here too the impersonal is found to be the most direct liberating force; it is through a wide egoless impersonality that one can become a free worker and a divine creator. It is not surprising that the overwhelming power of this experience from the impersonal pole of the Duality should have moved the sages to declare this to be the one way and an impersonal Superconscience to be the sole truth of the Eternal.

But still to the seeker standing at the opposite pole of the Duality another line of experience appears which justifies an intuition deeply-seated behind the heart and in our very life-force, that personality, like consciousness, life, soul, is not a brief-lived stranger in an impersonal Eternity, but contains the very meaning of existence. This fine flower of the cosmic Energy carries in it a forecast of the aim and a hint of the very motive of the universal labour. As an occult vision opens in him, he becomes aware of worlds behind in which consciousness and personality hold an enormous place and assume a premier value; even here in the material world to this occult vision the inconscience of Matter fills with a secret pervading consciousness, its inanimation harbours a vibrant life, its mechanism is the device of an indwelling Intelligence, God and soul are everywhere. Above all stands an infinite conscious Being who is variously self-expressed in all these worlds; impersonality is only a first means of that expression. It is a field of principles and forces, an equal basis of manifestation; but these forces express themselves through beings, have conscious spirits at their head and are the emanation of a One Conscious Being who is their source. A multiple innumerable personality expressing that One is the very sense and central aim of the manifestation and if now personality seems to be narrow, fragmentary, restrictive, it is only because it has not opened to its source or flowered into its own divine truth and fullness packing itself with the universal and the infinite. Thus the world-creation is no more an illusion, a fortuitous mechanism, a play that need not have happened, a flux without consequence; it is an intimate dynamism of the conscious and living Eternal.

This extreme opposition of view from the two poles of one Existence creates no fundamental difficulty for the seeker of the integral Yoga; for his whole experience has shown him the necessity of these double terms and their currents of Energy, negative and positive in relation to each other, for the manifestation of what is within the one Existence. For himself Personality and Impersonality have been the two wings of his spiritual ascension and he has the prevision that he will reach a height where their helpful interaction will pass into a fusion of their powers and disclose the integral Reality and release into action the original force of the Divine. Not only in the fundamental Aspects but in all the working of his sadhana he has felt their double truth and mutually complementary working. An impersonal Presence has dominated from above or penetrated and occupied his nature; a Light descending has suffused his mind, life-power, the very cells of his body, illumined them with knowledge, revealed him to himself down to his most disguised and unsuspected movements, exposing, purifying, destroying or brilliantly changing all that belonged to the Ignorance. A Force has poured into him in currents or like a sea, worked in his being and all its members, dissolved, new-made, reshaped, transfigured everywhere. A Bliss has invaded him and shown that it can make suffering and sorrow impossible and turn pain itself into divine pleasure. A Love without limits has joined him to all creatures or revealed to him a world of inseparable intimacy and unspeakable sweetness and beauty and begun to impose its law of perfection and its ecstasy even amidst the disharmony of terrestrial life. A spiritual Truth and Right have convicted the good and evil of this world of imperfection or of falsehood and unveiled a supreme good and its clue of subtle harmony and its sublimation of action and feeling and knowledge. But behind all these and in them he has felt a Divinity who is all these things, a Bringer of Light, a Guide and All-Knower, a Master of Force, a Giver of Bliss, Friend, Helper, Father, Mother, Playmate in the world-game, an absolute Master of his being, his soul's Beloved and Lover. All relations known to human personality are there in the soul's contact with the Divine; but they rise towards superhuman levels and compel him towards a divine nature.

It is an integral knowledge that is being sought, an integral force, a total amplitude of union with the All and Infinite behind existence. For the seeker of the integral Yoga no single experience, no one Divine Aspect,—however overwhelming to the human mind, sufficient for its capacity, easily accepted as the sole or the ultimate reality,—can figure as the exclusive truth of the Eternal. For him the experience of the Divine Oneness carried to its extreme is more deeply embraced and amply fathomed by following out to the full the experience of the Divine Multiplicity. All that is true behind polytheism as well as behind monotheism falls within the scope of his seeking; but he passes beyond their superficial sense to human mind to grasp their mystic truth in the Divine. He sees what is aimed at by the jarring sects and philosophies and accepts each facet of the Reality in its own place, but rejects their narrownesses and errors and proceeds farther till he discovers the One Truth that binds them together. The reproach of anthropomorphism and anthropolatry cannot deter him,—for he sees them to be prejudices of the ignorant and arrogant reasoning intelligence, the abstracting mind turning on itself in its own cramped circle. If human relations as practised now by man are full of smallness and perversity and ignorance, yet are they disfigured shadows of something in the Divine and by turning them to the Divine he finds that of which they are a shadow and brings it down for manifestation in life. It is through the human exceeding itself and opening itself to a supreme plenitude that the Divine must manifest itself here, since that comes inevitably in the course and process of the spiritual evolution, and therefore he will not despise or blind himself to the Godhead because it is lodged in a human body, *mānuṣīm˙ tanum āśritam* . Beyond the limited human conception of God, he will pass to the one divine Eternal, but also he will meet him in the faces of the Gods, his cosmic personalities supporting the World-Play, detect him behind the mask of the Vibhutis, embodied World-Forces or human Leaders, reverence and obey him in the Guru, worship him in the Avatar. This will be to him his exceeding good fortune if he can meet one who has realised or is becoming That which he seeks for and can by opening to it in this vessel of its manifestation himself realise it. For that is the most palpable sign of the growing fulfilment, the promise of the great mystery of the progressive Descent into Matter which is the secret sense of the material creation and the justification of terrestrial existence.

Thus reveals himself to the seeker in the progress of the sacrifice the Lord of the sacrifice. At any point this revelation can begin; in any aspect the Master of the Work can take up the work in him and more and more press upon him and it for the unfolding of his presence. In time all the Aspects disclose themselves, separate, combine, fuse, are unified together. At the end there shines through it all the supreme integral Reality, unknowable to Mind which is part of the Ignorance, but knowable because self-aware in the light of a spiritual consciousness and a supramental knowledge.

~

This revelation of a highest Truth or a highest Being, Consciousness, Power, Bliss and Love, impersonal and personal at once and so taking up both sides of our own being,—since in us also is the ambiguous meeting of a Person and a mass of impersonal principles and forces,—is at once the first aim and the condition of the ultimate achievement of the sacrifice. The achievement itself takes the shape of a union of our own existence with That which is thus made manifest to our vision and experience, and the union has a threefold character. There is a union in spiritual essence, by identity; there is a union by the indwelling of our soul in this highest Being and Consciousness; there is a dynamic union of likeness or oneness of nature between That and our instrumental being here. The first is the liberation from the Ignorance and identification with the Real and Eternal, *mokṣa, sāyujya*, which is the characteristic aim of the Yoga of Knowledge. The second, the dwelling of the soul with or in the Divine, *sāmīpya, sālokya*, is the intense hope of all Yoga of love and beatitude. The third, identity in nature, likeness to the Divine, to be perfect as That is perfect, is the high intention of all Yoga of power and perfection or of divine works and service. The combined completeness of the three together, founded here on a multiple Unity of the self-manifesting Divine, is the complete result of the integral Yoga, the goal of its triple Path and the fruit of its triple sacrifice.

A union by identity may be ours, a liberation and change of our substance of being into that supreme Spirit-substance, of our consciousness into that divine Consciousness, of our soul-state into that ecstasy of spiritual beatitude or that calm eternal bliss of existence. A luminous indwelling in the Divine can be attained by us secure against any fall or exile into this lower consciousness of the darkness and the Ignorance, the soul ranging freely and firmly in its own natural world of light and joy and freedom and oneness. And since this is not merely to be attained in some other existence beyond but pursued and discovered here also, it can only be by a descent, by a bringing down of the Divine Truth, by the establishment here of the soul's native world of light, joy, freedom, oneness. A union of our instrumental being no less than of our soul and spirit must change our imperfect nature into the very likeness and image of Divine Nature; it must put off the blind, marred, mutilated, discordant movements of the Ignorance and put on the inherence of that light, peace, bliss, harmony, universality, mystery, purity, perfection; it must convert itself into a receptacle of divine knowledge, an instrument of divine Will-Power and Force of Being, a channel of divine Love, Joy and Beauty. This is the transformation to be effected, an integral transformation of all that we now are or seem to be, by the joining—Yoga—of the finite being in Time with the Eternal and Infinite.

All this difficult result can become possible only if there is an immense conversion, a total reversal of our consciousness, a supernormal entire transfiguration of the nature. There must be an ascension of the whole being, an ascension of spirit chained here and trammelled by its instruments and its environment to sheer Spirit free above, an ascension of soul towards some blissful Super-soul, an ascension of mind towards some luminous Supermind, an ascension of life towards some vast Super-life, an ascension of our very physicality to join its origin in some pure and plastic spirit-substance. And this cannot be a single swift up-soaring but, like the ascent of the sacrifice described in the Veda, a climbing from peak to peak in which from each summit one looks up to the much more that has still to be done. At the same time there must be a descent too to affirm below what we have gained above: on each height we conquer we have to turn to bring down its power and its illumination into the lower mortal movement; the discovery of the Light for ever radiant on high must correspond with the release of the same Light secret below in every part down to the deepest caves of subconscient Nature. And this pilgrimage of ascension and this descent for the labour of transformation must be inevitably a battle, a long war with ourselves and with opposing forces around us which, while it lasts, may well seem interminable. For all our old obscure and ignorant nature will contend repeatedly and obstinately with the transforming Influence, supported in its lagging unwillingness or its stark resistance by most of the established forces of environing universal Nature; the powers and principalities and the ruling beings of the Ignorance will not easily give up their empire.

At first there may have to be a prolonged, often tedious and painful period of preparation and purification of all our being till it is ready and fit for an opening to a greater Truth and Light or to the Divine Influence and

Presence. Even when centrally fitted, prepared, open already, it will still be long before all our movements of mind, life and body, all the multiple and conflicting members and elements of our personality consent or, consenting, are able to bear the difficult and exacting process of the transformation. And hardest of all, even if all in us is willing, is the struggle we shall have to carry through against the universal forces attached to the present unstable creation when we seek to make the final supramental conversion and reversal of consciousness by which the Divine Truth must be established in us in its plenitude and not merely what they would more readily permit, an illumined Ignorance.

It is for this that a surrender and submission to That which is beyond us enabling the full and free working of its Power is indispensable. As that self-giving progresses, the work of the sacrifice becomes easier and more powerful and the prevention of the opposing Forces loses much of its strength, impulsion and substance. Two inner changes help most to convert what now seems difficult or impracticable into a thing possible and even sure. There takes place a coming to the front of some secret inmost soul within which was veiled by the restless activity of the mind, by the turbulence of our vital impulses and by the obscurity of the physical consciousness, the three powers which in their confused combination we now call our self. There will come about as a result a less impeded growth of a Divine Presence at the centre with its liberating Light and effective Force and an irradiation of it into all the conscious and subconscious ranges of our nature. These are the two signs, one marking our completed conversion and consecration to the great Quest, the other the final acceptance by the Divine of our sacrifice.

CHAPTER V. THE ASCENT OF THE SACRIFICE–1

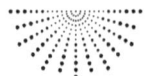

THE WORKS OF KNOWLEDGE — THE PSYCHIC BEING

THIS THEN is in its foundations the integral knowledge of the Supreme and Infinite to whom we offer our sacrifice, and this the nature of the sacrifice itself in its triple character,—a sacrifice of works, a sacrifice of love and adoration, a sacrifice of knowledge. For even when we speak of the sacrifice of works by itself, we do not mean the offering only of our outward acts, but of all that is active and dynamic in us; our internal movements no less than our external doings are to be consecrated on the one altar. The inner heart of all work that is made into a sacrifice is a labour of self-discipline and self-perfection by which we can hope to become conscious and luminous with a Light from above poured into all our movements of mind, heart, will, sense, life and body. An increasing light of divine consciousness will make us close in soul and one by identity in our inmost being and spiritual substance with the Master of the world-sacrifice,—the supreme object of existence proposed by the ancient Vedanta; but also it will tend to make us one in our becoming by resemblance to the Divine in our nature, the mystic sense of the symbol of sacrifice in the sealed speech of the seers of the Veda.

But if this is to be the character of the rapid evolution from a mental to a spiritual being contemplated by the integral Yoga, a question arises full of many perplexities but of great dynamic importance. How are we to deal with life and works as they now are, with the activities proper to our still unchanged human nature? An ascension towards a greater consciousness, an occupation of our mind, life and body by its powers has been accepted as the outstanding object of the Yoga: but still life here, not some other-life elsewhere, is proposed as the immediate field of the action of the Spirit,—a transformation, not an annihilation of our instrumental being and nature.

What then becomes of the present activities of our being, activities of the mind turned towards knowledge and the expression of knowledge, activities of our emotional and sensational parts, activities of outward conduct, creation, production, the will turned towards mastery over men, things, life, the world, the forces of Nature? Are they to be abandoned and to be replaced by some other way of living in which a spiritualised consciousness can find its true expression and figure? Are they to be maintained as they are in their outward appearance, but transformed by an inner spirit in the act or enlarged in scope and liberated into new forms by a reversal of consciousness such as was seen on earth when man took up the vital activities of the animal to mentalise and extend and transfigure them by the infusion of reason, thinking will, refined emotion, an organised intelligence? Or is there to be an abandonment in part, a preservation only of such of them as can bear a spiritual change and, for the rest, the creation of a new life expressive, in its form no less than in its inspiration and motive-force, of the unity, wideness, peace, joy and harmony of the liberated spirit? It is this problem most of all that has exercised the minds of those who have tried to trace the paths that lead from the human to the Divine in the long journey of the Yoga.

Every kind of solution has been offered from the entire abandonment of works and life, so far as that is physically possible, to the acceptance of life as it is but with a new spirit animating and uplifting its movements, in appearance the same as they were but changed in the spirit behind them and therefore in their inner significance. The extreme solution insisted on by the world-shunning ascetic or the inward-turned ecstatical and self-oblivious mystic is evidently foreign to the purpose of an integral Yoga,— for if we are to realise the Divine in the world, it cannot be done by leaving aside the world-action and action itself altogether. At a less high pitch it was laid down by the religious mind in ancient times that one should keep only such actions as are in their nature part of the seeking, service or cult of the Divine and such others as are attached to these or, in addition, those that are indispensable to the ordinary setting of life but done in a religious spirit and according to the injunctions of traditional religion and Scripture. But this is too formalist a rule for the fulfilment of the free spirit in works, and it is besides professedly no more than a provisional solution for tiding over the transition from life in the world to a life in the Beyond which still remains the sole ultimate purpose. An integral Yoga must lean rather to the catholic injunction of the Gita that even the liberated soul, living in the Truth, should still do all the works of life so that the plan of the universal evolution under a secret divine leading may not languish or suffer. But if all works are to be done with the same forms and on the same lines as they are now done in the Ignorance, our gain is only inward and our life is in danger of becoming the dubious and ambiguous formula of an inner Light doing the works of an outer Twilight, the perfect Spirit expressing itself in a mould of imperfection foreign to its own divine nature. If no better can be done for a time,—and during a long period of transition something like this does inevitably happen,—then so it must remain till things are ready and the spirit within is powerful enough to impose its own forms on the life of the body and the world outside; but this can be accepted only as a transitional stage and not as our soul's ideal or the ultimate goal of the passage.

For the same reason the ethical solution is insufficient; for an ethical rule merely puts a bit in the mouth of the wild horses of Nature and exercises over them a difficult and partial control, but it has no power to transform Nature so that she may move in a secure freedom fulfilling the intuitions that proceed from a divine self-knowledge. At best its method is to lay down limits, to coerce the devil, to put the wall of a relative and very doubtful safety around us. This or some similar device of self-protection may be necessary for a time whether in ordinary life or in Yoga; but in Yoga it can only be the mark of a transition. A fundamental transformation and a pure wideness of spiritual life are the aim before us and, if we are to reach it, we must find a deeper solution, a surer supra-ethical dynamic principle. To be spiritual within, ethical in the outside life, this is the ordinary religious solution, but it is a compromise; the spiritualisation of both the inward being and the outward life and not a compromise between life and the spirit is the goal of which we are the seekers. Nor can the human confusion of values which obliterates the distinction between spiritual and moral and even claims that the moral is the only true spiritual element in our nature be of any use to us; for ethics is a mental control, and the limited erring mind is not and cannot be the free and ever-luminous spirit. It is equally impossible to accept the gospel that makes life the one aim, takes its elements fundamentally as they are and only calls in a half-spiritual or pseudo-spiritual light to flush and embellish it. Inadequate too is the very frequent attempt at a misalliance between the vital and the spiritual, a mystic experience within with an aestheticised intellectual and sensuous Paganism or exalted hedonism outside leaning upon it and satisfying itself in the glow of a spiritual sanction; for this too is a precarious and never successful compromise and it is as far from the divine Truth and its integrality as the puritanic opposite. These are all stumbling solutions of the fallible human mind groping for a transaction between the high spiritual summits and the lower pitch of the ordinary mind-motives and life-motives. Whatever partial truth may be hidden behind them, that truth can only be accepted when it has been raised to the spiritual level, tested in the supreme Truth-consciousness and extricated from the soil and error of the Ignorance.

In sum, it may be safely affirmed that no solution offered can be anything but provisional until a supramental Truth-consciousness is reached by which the appearances of things are put in their place and their essence revealed and that in them which derives straight from the spiritual essence. In the meanwhile our only safety is to find a guiding law of spiritual experience—or else to liberate a light within that can lead us on the way until that greater direct Truth-consciousness is reached above us or born within us. For all else in us that is only outward, all that is not a spiritual sense or seeing, the constructions, representations or conclusions of the intellect, the suggestions or instigations of the life-force, the positive necessities of physical things are sometimes half-lights, sometimes false lights that can at best only serve for a while or serve a little and for the rest either detain or confuse us. The guiding law of spiritual experience can only come by an opening of human consciousness to the Divine Consciousness; there must be the power to receive in us the working and command and dynamic presence of the Divine Shakti and surrender ourselves to her control; it is that surrender and that control which bring the guidance. But the surrender is not sure, there is no absolute certitude of the guidance so long as we are besieged by mind formations and life impulses and instigations of ego which may easily betray us into the hands of a false experience. This danger can only be countered by the opening of a now nine-tenths concealed inmost soul or psychic being that is already there but not commonly active within us. That is the inner light we must liberate; for the light of this inmost soul is our one sure illumination so long as we walk still amidst the siege of the Ignorance and the Truth-consciousness has not taken up the entire control of our Godward endeavour. The working of the Divine Force in us under the conditions of the transition and the light of the psychic being turning us always towards a conscious and seeing obedience to that higher impulsion and away from the demands and instigations of the Forces of the Ignorance, these between them create an ever progressive inner law of our action which continues till the spiritual and supramental can be established in our nature. In the transition there may well be a period in which we take up all life and action and offer them to the Divine for purification, change and deliverance of the truth within them, another period in which we draw back and build a spiritual wall around us admitting through its gates only such activities as consent to undergo the law of the spiritual transformation, a third in which a free and all-embracing action, but with new forms fit for the utter truth of the Spirit, can again be made possible. These things, however, will be decided by no mental rule but in the light of the soul within us and by the ordaining force and progressive guidance of the Divine Power that secretly or overtly first impels, then begins clearly to control and order and finally takes up the whole burden of the Yoga.

In accordance with the triple character of the sacrifice we may divide works too into a triple order, the works of Knowledge, the works of Love, the works of the Will-in-Life, and see how this more plastic spiritual rule applies to each province and effects the transition from the lower to the higher nature.

~

It is natural from the point of view of the Yoga to divide into two categories the activities of the human mind in its pursuit of knowledge. There is the supreme supra-intellectual knowledge which concentrates itself on the discovery of the One and Infinite in its transcendence or tries to penetrate by intuition, contemplation, direct inner contact into the ultimate truths behind the appearances of Nature; there is the lower science which diffuses itself in an outward knowledge of phenomena, the disguises of the One and Infinite as it appears to us in or through the more exterior forms of the world-manifestation around us. These two, an upper and a lower hemisphere, in the form of them constructed or conceived by men within the mind's ignorant limits, have even there separated themselves, as they developed, with some sharpness.... Philosophy, sometimes spiritual or at least intuitive, sometimes abstract and intellectual, sometimes intellectualising spiritual experience or supporting with a logical apparatus the discoveries of the spirit, has claimed always to take the fixation of ultimate Truth as its province. But even when it did not separate itself on rarefied metaphysical heights from the knowledge that belongs to the practical world and the pursuit of ephemeral objects, intellectual Philosophy by its habit of abstraction has seldom been a power for life. It has been sometimes powerful for high speculation, pursuing mental Truth for its own sake without any ulterior utility or object, sometimes for a subtle gymnastic of the mind in a mistily bright cloud-land of words and ideas, but it has walked or acrobatised far from the more tangible realities of existence. Ancient Philosophy in Europe was more dynamic, but only for the few; in India in its more spiritualised forms, it strongly influenced but without transforming the life of the race.... Religion did not attempt, like Philosophy, to live alone on the heights; its aim was rather to take hold of man's parts of life even more than his parts of mind and draw them Godwards; it professed to build a bridge between spiritual Truth and the vital and material human existence; it strove to subordinate and reconcile the lower to the higher, make life serviceable to God, Earth obedient to Heaven. It has to be admitted that too often this necessary effort had the opposite result of making Heaven a sanction for Earth's desires; for, continually, the religious idea has been turned into an excuse for the worship and service of the human ego. Religion, leaving constantly its little shining core of spiritual experience, has lost itself in the obscure mass of its ever extending ambiguous compromises with life: in attempting to satisfy the thinking mind, it more often succeeded in oppressing or fettering it with a mass of theological dogmas; while seeking to net the human heart, it fell itself into pits of pietistic emotionalism and sensationalism; in the act of annexing the vital nature of man to dominate it, it grew itself vitiated and fell a prey to all the fanaticism, homicidal fury, savage or harsh turn for oppression, pullulating falsehood, obstinate attachment to ignorance to which that vital nature is prone; its desire to draw the physical in man towards God betrayed it into chaining itself to ecclesiastic mechanism, hollow ceremony and lifeless ritual. The corruption of the best produced the worst by that strange chemistry of the power of life which generates evil out of good even as it can also generate good out of evil. At the same time in a vain effort at self-defence against this downward gravitation, Religion was driven to cut existence into two by a division of knowledge, works, art, life itself into two opposite categories, the spiritual and the worldly, religious and mundane, sacred and profane; but this defensive distinction itself became conventional and artificial and aggravated rather than healed the disease.... On their side Science and Art and the knowledge of Life, although at first they served or lived in the shadow of Religion, ended by emancipating themselves, became estranged or hostile, or have even recoiled with indifference, contempt or scepticism from what seem to them the cold, barren and distant or unsubstantial and illusory heights of unreality to which metaphysical Philosophy and Religion aspire. For a time the divorce has been as complete as the one-sided intolerance of the human mind could make it and threatened even to end in a complete extinction of all attempt at a higher or a more spiritual knowledge. Yet even in the earthward life a higher knowledge is indeed the one thing that is throughout needful, and without it the lower sciences and pursuits, however fruitful, however rich, free, miraculous in the abundance of their results, become easily a sacrifice offered without due order and to false gods; corrupting, hardening in the end the heart of man, limiting his mind's horizons, they confine in a stony material imprisonment or lead to a final baffling incertitude and disillusionment. A sterile agnosticism awaits us above the brilliant phosphorescence of a half-knowledge that is still the Ignorance.

    A Yoga turned towards an all-embracing realisation of the Supreme will not despise the works or even the dreams, if dreams they are, of the Cosmic Spirit or shrink from the splendid toil and many-sided victory which he has assigned to himself in the human creature. But its first condition for this liberality is that our works in the world too must be part of the sacrifice offered to the Highest and to none else, to the Divine Shakti and to no other Power, in the right spirit and with the right knowledge, by the free soul and not by the hypnotised bondslave of material Nature. If a division of works has to be made, it is between those that are nearest to the heart of the sacred flame and those that are least touched or illumined by it because they are more at a distance, or between the fuel that burns strongly and brightly and the logs that if too thickly heaped on the altar may impede the ardour of the fire by their rather damp, heavy and diffused abundance. But, otherwise, apart from this division, all activities of knowledge that seek after or express Truth are in themselves rightful materials for a complete offering; none ought necessarily to be excluded from the wide framework of the divine life. The mental and physical sciences which examine into the laws and forms and processes of things, those which concern the life of men and animals, the social, political, linguistic and historical and those which seek to know and control the labours and activities by which man subdues and utilises his world and environment, and the noble and beautiful Arts which are at once work and knowledge,—for every well-made and significant poem, picture, statue or building is an act of creative knowledge, a living discovery of the consciousness, a figure of Truth, a dynamic form of mental and vital self-expression or world-expression,—all that seeks, all that finds, all that voices or figures is a realisation of something of the play of the Infinite and to that extent can be made a means of God-realisation or of divine formation. But the Yogin has to see that it is no longer done as part of an ignorant mental life; it can be accepted by him only if by the feeling, the remembrance, the dedication within it, it is turned into a movement of the spiritual consciousness and becomes a part of its vast grasp of comprehensive illuminating knowledge.

For all must be done as a sacrifice, all activities must have the One Divine for their object and the heart of their meaning. The Yogin's aim in the sciences that make for knowledge should be to discover and understand the workings of the Divine Consciousness-Puissance in man and creatures and things and forces, her creative significances, her execution of the mysteries, the symbols in which she arranges the manifestation. The Yogin's aim in the practical sciences, whether mental and physical or occult and psychic, should be to enter into the ways of the Divine and his processes, to know the materials and means for the work given to us so that we may use that knowledge for a conscious and faultless expression of the spirit's mastery, joy and self-fulfilment. The Yogin's aim in the Arts should not be a mere aesthetic, mental or vital gratification, but, seeing the Divine everywhere, worshipping it with a revelation of the meaning of its own works, to express that One Divine in ideal forms, the One Divine in principles and forces, the One Divine in gods and men and creatures and objects. The theory that sees an intimate connection between religious aspiration and the truest and greatest Art is in essence right; but we must substitute for the mixed and doubtful religious motive a spiritual aspiration, vision, interpreting experience. For the wider and more comprehensive the seeing, the more it contains in itself the sense of the hidden Divine in humanity and in all things and rises beyond a superficial religiosity into the spiritual life, the more luminous, flexible, deep and powerful will the Art be that springs from that high motive. The Yogin's distinction from other men is this that he lives in a higher and vaster spiritual consciousness; all his work of knowledge or creation must then spring from there: it must not be made in the mind,—for it is a greater truth and vision than mental man's that he has to express or rather that presses to express itself through him and mould his works, not for his personal satisfaction, but for a divine purpose.

At the same time the Yogin who knows the Supreme is not subject to any need or compulsion in these activities; for to him they are neither a duty nor a necessary occupation for the mind nor a high amusement, nor imposed even by the loftiest human purpose. He is not attached, bound and limited by any nor has he any personal motive of fame, greatness or personal satisfaction in these works; he can leave or pursue them as the Divine in him wills, but he need not otherwise abandon them in his pursuit of the higher integral knowledge. He will do these things just as the supreme Power acts and creates, for a certain spiritual joy in creation and expression or to help in the holding together and right ordering or leading of this world of God's workings. The Gita teaches that the man of knowledge shall by his way of life give to those who have not yet the spiritual consciousness, the love and habit of *all* works and not only of actions recognised as pious, religious or ascetic in their character; he should not draw men away from the world-action by his example. For the world must proceed in its great upward aspiring; men and nations must not be led to fall away from even an ignorant activity into a worse ignorance of inaction or to sink down into that miserable disintegration and tendency of dissolution which comes upon communities and peoples when there predominates the tamasic principle, the principle whether of obscure confusion and error or of weariness and inertia. "For I too," says the Lord in the Gita, "have no need to do works, since there is nothing I have not or must yet gain for myself; yet I do works in the world: for if I did not do works, all laws would fall into confusion, the worlds would sink towards chaos and I would be the destroyer of these peoples." The spiritual life does not need, for its purity, to destroy interest in all things except the Inexpressible or to cut at the roots of the Sciences, the Arts and Life. It may well be one of the effects of an integral spiritual knowledge and activity to lift them out of their limitations, substitute for our mind's ignorant, limited, tepid or trepidant pleasure in them a free, intense and uplifting urge of delight and supply a new source of creative spiritual power and illumination by which they can be carried more swiftly and profoundly towards their absolute light in knowledge and their yet undreamed possibilities and most dynamic energy of content and form and practice. The one thing needful must be pursued first and always; but all things else come with it as its outcome and have not so much to be added to us as recovered and reshaped in its self-light and as portions of its self-expressive force.

This then is the true relation between divine and human knowledge; it is not a separation into disparate fields, sacred and profane, that is the heart of the difference, but the character of the consciousness behind the working. All is human knowledge that proceeds from the ordinary mental consciousness interested in the outside or upper layers of things, in process, in phenomena for their own sake or for the sake of some surface utility or mental or vital satisfaction of Desire or of the Intelligence. But the same activity of knowledge can become part of the Yoga if it proceeds from the spiritual or spiritualising consciousness which seeks and finds in all that it surveys or penetrates the presence of the timeless Eternal and the ways of manifestation of the Eternal in Time. It is evident that the need of a concentration indispensable for the transition out of the Ignorance may make it necessary for the seeker to gather together his energies and focus them only on that which will help the transition and to leave aside or subordinate for the time all that is not directly turned towards the one object. He may find that this or that pursuit of human knowledge with which he was accustomed to deal by the surface power of the mind still brings him by reason of this tendency or habit out of the depths to the surface or down from the heights which he has climbed or is nearing to lower levels. These activities then may have to be intermitted or put aside until, secure in a higher consciousness, he is able to turn its powers on all the mental fields; then, subjected to that light or taken up into it, they are turned, by the transformation of his consciousness, into a province of the spiritual and divine. All that cannot be so transformed or refuses to be part of a divine consciousness he will abandon without hesitation, but not from any preconceived prejudgment of its unfitness or its incapacity to be an element of the new inner life. There can be no fixed mental test or principle for these things; he will therefore follow no unalterable rule, but accept or repel an activity of the mind according to his feeling, insight or experience until the greater Power and Light are there to turn their unerring scrutiny on all that is below and choose or reject their material out of what the human evolution has prepared for the divine labour.

How precisely or by what stages this progression and change will take place must depend on the form, need and powers of the individual nature. In the spiritual domain the essence is always one, but there is yet an infinite variety and, at any rate in the integral Yoga, the rigidity of a strict and precise mental rule is seldom applicable; for, even when they walk in the same direction, no two natures proceed on exactly the same lines, in the same series of steps or with quite identical stages of their progress. It may yet be said that a logical succession of the states of progress would be very much in this order. First, there is a large turning in which all the natural mental activities proper to the individual nature are taken up or referred to a higher standpoint and dedicated by the soul in us, the psychic being, the priest of the sacrifice, to the divine service; next, there is an attempt at an ascent of the being and a bringing down of the Light and Power proper to some new height of consciousness gained by its upward effort into the whole action of the knowledge. Here there may be a strong concentration on the inward central change of the consciousness and an abandonment of a large part of the outward-going mental life or else its relegation to a small and subordinate place. At different stages it or parts of it may be taken up again from time to time to see how far the new inner psychic and spiritual consciousness can be brought into its movements; but that compulsion of the temperament or the nature which in human beings necessitates one kind of activity or another and makes it seem almost an indispensable portion of the existence, will diminish and eventually no attachment will be left, no lower compulsion or driving force felt anywhere. Only the Divine will matter, the Divine alone will be the one need of the whole being; if there is any compulsion to activity it will be not that of implanted desire or of force of Nature, but the luminous driving of some greater Consciousness-Force which is becoming more and more the sole motive power of the whole existence. On the other hand, it is possible at any period of the inner spiritual progress that one may experience an extension rather than a restriction of the activities; there may be an opening of new capacities of mental creation and new provinces of knowledge by the miraculous touch of the Yoga-Shakti. Aesthetic feeling, the power of artistic creation in one field or many fields together, talent or genius of literary expression, a faculty of metaphysical thinking, any power of eye or ear or hand or mind-power may awaken where none was apparent before. The Divine within may throw these latent riches out from the depths in which they were hidden or a Force from above may pour down its energies to equip the instrumental nature for the activity or the creation of which it is meant to be a channel or a builder. But, whatever may be the method or the course of development chosen by the hidden Master of the Yoga, the common culmination of this stage is the growing consciousness of him alone as the mover, decider, shaper of all the movements of the mind and all the activities of knowledge.

There are two signs of the transformation of the seeker's mind of knowledge and works of knowledge from the process of the Ignorance to the process of a liberated consciousness working partly, then wholly in the light of the Spirit. There is first a central change of the consciousness and a growing direct experience, vision, feeling of the Supreme and the cosmic existence, the Divine in itself and the Divine in all things; the mind will be taken up into a growing preoccupation with this first and foremost and will feel itself heightening, widening into a more and more illumined means of expression of the one fundamental knowledge. But also the central Consciousness in its turn will take up more and more the outer mental activities of knowledge and turn them into a parcel of itself or an annexed province; it will infuse into them its more authentic movement and make a more and more spiritualised and illumined mind its instrument in these surface fields, its new conquests, as well as in its own deeper spiritual empire. And this will be the second sign, the sign of a certain completion and perfection, that the Divine himself has become the Knower and all the inner movements, including the activities of what was once a purely human mental action, have become his field of knowledge. There will be less and less individual choice, opinion, preference, less and less of intellectualisation, mental weaving, cerebral galley-slave labour; a Light within will see all that has to be seen, know all that has to be known, develop, create, organise. It will be the Inner Knower who will do in the liberated and universalised mind of the individual the works of an all-comprehending knowledge.

These two changes are the signs of a first effectuation in which the activities of the mental nature are lifted up, spiritualised, widened, universalised, liberated, led to a consciousness of their true purpose as an instrumentation of the Divine creating and developing its manifestation in the temporal universe. But this cannot be the whole scope of the transformation; for it is not in these limits that the integral seeker can cease from his ascension or confine the widening of his nature. For, if it were so, knowledge would still remain a working of the mind, liberated, universalised, spiritualised, but still, as all mind must be, comparatively restricted, relative, imperfect in the very essence of its dynamism; it would reflect luminously great constructions of Truth, but not move in the domain where Truth is authentic, direct, sovereign and native. There is an ascension still to be made from this height, by which the spiritualised mind will exceed itself and transmute into a supramental power of knowledge. Already in the process of spiritualisation it will have begun to pass out of the brilliant poverty of the human intellect; it will mount successively into the pure broad reaches of a higher mind, and next into the gleaming belts of a still greater free Intelligence illumined with a Light from above. At this point it will begin to feel more freely, admit with a less mixed response the radiant beginnings of an Intuition, not illumined, but luminous in itself, true in itself, no longer entirely mental and therefore subjected to the abundant intrusion of error. Here too is not an end, for it must rise beyond into the very domain of that untruncated Intuition, the first direct light from the self-awareness of essential Being and, beyond it, attain that from which this light comes. For there is an Overmind behind Mind, a Power more original and dynamic which supports Mind, sees it as a diminished radiation from itself, uses it as a transmitting belt of passage downward or an instrument for the creations of the Ignorance. The last step of the ascension would be the surpassing of Overmind itself or its return into its own still greater origin, its conversion into the supramental light of the Divine

Gnosis. For there in the supramental Light is the seat of a divine Truth-consciousness that has native in it, as no other consciousness below it can have, the power to organise the works of a Truth which is no longer tarnished by the shadow of the cosmic Inconscience and Ignorance. There to reach and thence to bring down a supramental dynamism that can transform the Ignorance is the distant but imperative supreme goal of the integral Yoga.

As the light of each of these higher powers is turned upon the human activities of knowledge, any distinction of sacred and profane, human and divine, begins more and more to fade until it is finally abolished as otiose; for whatever is touched and thoroughly penetrated by the Divine Gnosis is transfigured and becomes a movement of its own Light and Power, free from the turbidity and limitations of the lower intelligence. It is not a separation of some activities, but a transformation of them all by the change of the informing consciousness that is the way of liberation, an ascent of the sacrifice of knowledge to a greater and ever greater light and force. All the works of mind and intellect must be first heightened and widened, then illumined, lifted into the domain of a higher Intelligence, afterwards translated into workings of a greater non-mental Intuition, these again transformed into the dynamic outpourings of the Overmind radiance, and those transfigured into the full light and sovereignty of the supramental Gnosis. It is this that the evolution of consciousness in the world carries prefigured but latent in its seed and in the straining tense intention of its process; nor can that process, that evolution cease till it has evolved the instruments of a perfect in place of its now imperfect manifestation of the Spirit.

If knowledge is the widest power of the consciousness and its function is to free and illumine, yet love is the deepest and most intense and its privilege is to be the key to the most profound and secret recesses of the Divine Mystery. Man, because he is a mental being, is prone to give the highest importance to the thinking mind and its reason and will and to its way of approach and effectuation of Truth and, even, he is inclined to hold that there is no other. The heart with its emotions and incalculable movements is to the eye of his intellect an obscure, uncertain and often a perilous and misleading power which needs to be kept in control by the reason and the mental will and intelligence. And yet there is in the heart or behind it a profounder mystic light which, if not what we call intuition,—for that, though not of the mind, yet descends through the mind,—has yet a direct touch upon Truth and is nearer to the Divine than the human intellect in its pride of knowledge. According to the ancient teaching the seat of the immanent Divine, the hidden Purusha, is in the mystic heart,—the secret heart-cave, *hṛdaye guhāyām*, as the Upanishads put it,—and, according to the experience of many Yogins, it is from its depths that there comes the voice or the breath of the inner oracle.

This ambiguity, these opposing appearances of depth and blindness are created by the double character of the human emotive being. For there is in front in man a heart of vital emotion similar to the animal's, if more variously developed; its emotions are governed by egoistic passion, blind instinctive affections and all the play of the life-impulses with their imperfections, perversions, often sordid degradations,—a heart besieged and given over to the lusts, desires, wraths, intense or fierce demands or little greeds and mean pettinesses of an obscure and fallen life-force and debased by its slavery to any and every impulse. This mixture of the emotive heart and the sensational hungering vital creates in man a false soul of desire; it is this that is the crude and dangerous element which the reason rightly distrusts and feels a need to control, even though the actual control or rather coercion it succeeds in establishing over our raw and insistent vital nature remains always very uncertain and deceptive. But the true soul of man is not there; it is in the true invisible heart hidden in some luminous cave of the nature: there under some infiltration of the divine Light is our soul, a silent inmost being of which few are even aware; for if all have a soul, few are conscious of their true soul or feel its direct impulse. There dwells the little spark of the Divine which supports the obscure mass of our nature and around it grows the psychic being, the formed soul or the real Man within us. It is as this psychic being in him grows and the movements of the heart reflect its divinations and impulsions that man becomes more and more aware of his soul, ceases to be a superior animal and, awakening to glimpses of the godhead within him, admits more and more its intimations of a deeper life and consciousness and an impulse towards things divine. It is one of the decisive moments of the integral Yoga when this psychic being, liberated, brought out from the veil to the front, can pour the full flood of its divinations, seeings and impulsions on the mind, life and body of man and begins to prepare the upbuilding of divinity in the earthly nature.

As in the works of knowledge, so in dealing with the workings of the heart, we are obliged to make a preliminary distinction between two categories of movements, those that are either moved by the true soul or aid towards its liberation and rule in the nature and those that are turned to the satisfaction of the unpurified vital nature. But the distinctions ordinarily laid down in this sense are of little use for the deeper spiritual purpose of Yoga. Thus a division can be made between religious emotions and mundane feelings and it can be laid down as a rule of spiritual life that the religious emotions alone should be cultivated and all worldly feelings and passions must be rejected and fall away from our existence. This in practice would mean the religious life of the saint or devotee, alone within with the Divine or linked only to others in a common God-love or at the most pouring out the fountains of a sacred, religious or pietistic love on the world outside. But religious emotion itself is too constantly invaded by the turmoil and obscurity of the vital movements and it is often either crude or narrow or fanatical or mixed with movements that are not signs of the spirit's perfection. It is evident besides that even at the best an intense figure of sainthood clamped in rigid hieratic lines is quite other than the wide ideal of an integral Yoga. A larger psychic and emotional relation with God and the world, more deep and plastic in its essence, more wide and embracing in its movements, more capable of taking up in its sweep the whole of life, is imperative.

A wider formula has been provided by the secular mind of man of which the basis is the ethical sense; for it distinguishes between the emotions sanctioned by the ethical sense and those that are egoistic and selfishly common and mundane. It is the works of altruism, philanthropy, compassion, benevolence, humanitarianism, service, labour for the wellbeing of man and all creatures that are to be our ideal; to shuffle off the coil of egoism and grow into a soul of self-abnegation that lives only or mainly for others or for humanity as a whole is the way of man's inner evolution according to this doctrine. Or if this is too secular and mental to satisfy the whole of our being, since there is a deeper religious and spiritual note there that is left out of account by the humanitarian formula, a religio-ethical foundation can be provided for it—and such was indeed its original basis. To the inner worship of the Divine or the Supreme by the devotion of the heart or to the pursuit of the Ineffable by the seeking of a highest knowledge can be added a worship through altruistic works or a preparation through acts of love, of benevolence, of service to mankind or to those around us. It is indeed by the religio-ethical sense that the law of universal goodwill or universal compassion or of love and service to the neighbour, the Vedantic, the Buddhistic, the Christian ideal, was created; only by a sort of secular refrigeration extinguishing the fervour of the religious element in it could the humanitarian ideal disengage itself and become the highest plane of a secular system of mental and moral ethics. For in the religious system this law of works is a means that ceases when its object is accomplished or a side issue; it is a part of the cult by which one adores and seeks the Divinity or it is a penultimate step of the excision of self in the passage to Nirvana. In the secular ideal it is promoted into an object in itself; it becomes a sign of the moral perfection of the human being, or else it is a condition for a happier state of man upon earth, a better society, a more united life of the race. But none of these things satisfy the demand of the soul that is placed before us by the integral Yoga.

Altruism, philanthropy, humanitarianism, service are flowers of the mental consciousness and are at best the mind's cold and pale imitation of the spiritual flame of universal Divine Love. Not truly liberative from ego-sense, they widen it at most and give it a higher and larger satisfaction; impotent in practice to change man's vital life and nature, they only modify and palliate its action and daub over its unchanged egoistic essence. Or if they are intensely followed with an entire sincerity of the will, it is by an exaggerated amplification of one side of our nature; in that exaggeration there can be no clue for the full and perfect divine evolution of the many sides of our individualised being towards the universal and transcendent Eternal. Nor can the religio-ethical ideal be a sufficient guide, —for this is a compromise or compact of mutual concessions for mutual support between a religious urge which seeks to get a closer hold on earth by taking into itself the higher turns of ordinary human nature and an ethical urge which hopes to elevate itself out of its own mental hardness and dryness by some touch of a religious fervour. In making this compact religion lowers itself to the mental level and inherits the inherent imperfections of mind and its inability to convert and transform life. The mind is the sphere of the dualities and, just as it is impossible for it to achieve any absolute Truth but only truths relative or mixed with error, so it is impossible for it to achieve any absolute good; for moral good exists as a counterpart and corrective to evil and has evil always for its shadow, complement, almost its reason for existence. But the spiritual consciousness belongs to a higher than the mental plane and there the dualities cease; for there falsehood confronted with the truth by which it profited through a usurping falsification of it and evil faced by the good of which it was a perversion or a lurid substitute, are obliged to perish for want of sustenance and to cease. The integral Yoga, refusing to rely upon the fragile stuff of mental and moral ideals, puts its whole emphasis in this field on three central dynamic processes,—the development of the true soul or psychic being to take the place of the false soul of desire, the sublimation of human into divine love, the elevation of consciousness from its mental to its spiritual and supramental plane by whose power alone both the soul and the life-force can be utterly delivered from the veils and prevarications of the Ignorance.

It is the very nature of the soul or the psychic being to turn towards the divine Truth as the sunflower to the sun; it accepts and clings to all that is divine or progressing towards divinity, and draws back from all that is a perversion or a denial of it, from all that is false and undivine. Yet the soul is at first but a spark and then a little flame of godhead burning in the midst of a great darkness; for the most part it is veiled in its inner sanctum and to reveal itself it has to call on the mind, the life-force and the physical consciousness and persuade them, as best they can, to express it; ordinarily, it succeeds at most in suffusing their outwardness with its inner light and modifying with its purifying fineness their dark obscurities or their coarser mixture. Even when there is a formed psychic being able to express itself with some directness in life, it is still in all but a few a smaller portion of the being—"no bigger in the mass of the body than the thumb of a man" was the image used by the ancient seers—and it is not always able to prevail against the obscurity or ignorant smallness of the physical consciousness, the mistaken surenesses of the mind or the arrogance and vehemence of the vital nature. This soul is obliged to accept the human mental, emotive, sensational life as it is, its relations, its activities, its cherished forms and figures; it has to labour to disengage and increase the divine element in all this relative truth mixed with a continual falsifying error, this love turned to the uses of the animal body or the satisfaction of the vital ego, this life of an average manhood shot with rare and pale glimpses of godhead and the darker luridities of the demon and the brute. Unerring in the essence of its will, it is obliged often under the pressure of its instruments to submit to mistakes of action, wrong placement of feeling, wrong choice of person, errors in the exact form of its will, in the circumstances of its expression of the infallible inner ideal. Yet is there a divination within it which makes it a surer guide than the reason or than even the highest desire, and through apparent errors and stumblings its voice can still lead better than the precise intellect and the considering mental judgment. This voice of the soul is not what we call conscience—for that is only a mental and often conventional erring substitute; it is a deeper and more seldom heard call; yet to follow it when heard is wisest: even, it is better to wander at the call of one's soul than to go apparently straight with the reason and the outward moral mentor. But it is only when the life turns towards the Divine that the soul can truly come forward and impose its power on the outer members; for, itself a spark of the Divine, to grow in flame towards the Divine is its true life and its very reason of existence.

At a certain stage in the Yoga when the mind is sufficiently quieted and no longer supports itself at every step on the sufficiency of its mental certitudes, when the vital has been steadied and subdued and is no longer constantly insistent on its own rash will, demand and desire, when the physical has been sufficiently altered not to bury altogether the inner flame under the mass of its outwardness, obscurity or inertia, an inmost being, long hidden within and felt only in its rare influences, is able to come forward and illumine the rest and take up the lead of the Sadhana. Its character is a one-pointed orientation towards the Divine or the Highest, one-pointed and yet plastic in action and movement; it does not create a rigidity of direction like the one-pointed intellect or a bigotry of the regnant idea or impulse like the one-pointed vital force; it is at every moment and with a supple sureness that it points the way to the Truth, automatically distinguishes the right step from the false, extricates the divine or Godward movement from the clinging mixture of the undivine. Its action is like a searchlight showing up all that has to be changed in the nature; it has in it a flame of will insistent on perfection, on an alchemic transmutation of all the inner and outer existence. It sees the divine essence everywhere but rejects the mere mask and the disguising figure. It insists on Truth, on will and strength and mastery, on Joy and Love and Beauty, but on a Truth of abiding Knowledge that surpasses the mere practical momentary truth of the Ignorance, on an inward joy and not on mere vital pleasure,—for it prefers rather a purifying suffering and sorrow to degrading satisfactions,—on love winged upward and not tied to the stake of egoistic craving or with its feet sunk in the mire, on beauty restored to its priesthood of interpretation of the Eternal, on strength and will and mastery as instruments not of the ego but of the Spirit. Its will is for the divinisation of life, the expression through it of a higher Truth, its dedication to the Divine and the Eternal.

But the most intimate character of the psychic is its pressure towards the Divine through a sacred love, joy and oneness. It is a divine Love that it seeks most, it is the love of the Divine that is its spur, its goal, its star of Truth shining over the luminous cave of the nascent or the still obscure cradle of the new-born godhead within us. In the first long stage of its growth and immature existence it has leaned on earthly love, affection, tenderness, goodwill, compassion, benevolence, on all beauty and gentleness and fineness and light and strength and courage, on all that can help to refine and purify the grossness and commonness of human nature; but it knows how mixed are these human movements at their best and at their worst how fallen and stamped with the mark of ego and self-deceptive sentimental falsehood and the lower self profiting by the imitation of a soulmovement. At once, emerging, it is ready and eager to break all the old ties and imperfect emotional activities and replace them by a greater spiritual Truth of love and oneness. It may still admit the human forms and movements, but on condition that they are turned towards the One alone. It accepts only the ties that are helpful, the heart's and mind's reverence for the Guru, the union of the God-seekers, a spiritual compassion for this ignorant human and animal world and its peoples, the joy and happiness and satisfaction of beauty that comes from the perception of the Divine everywhere. It plunges the nature inward towards its meeting with the immanent Divine in the heart's secret centre and, while that call is there, no reproach of egoism, no mere outward summons of altruism or duty or philanthropy or service will deceive or divert it from its sacred longing and its obedience to the attraction of the Divinity within it. It lifts the being towards a transcendent Ecstasy and is ready to shed all the downward pull of the world from its wings in its uprising to reach the One Highest; but it calls down also this transcendent Love and Beatitude to deliver and transform this world of hatred and strife and division and darkness and jarring Ignorance. It opens to a universal Divine Love, a vast compassion, an intense and immense will for the good of all, for the embrace of the World-Mother enveloping or gathering to her her children, the divine Passion that has plunged into the night for the redemption of the world from the universal Inconscience. It is not attracted or misled by mental imitations or any vital misuse of these great deep-seated Truths of existence; it exposes them with its detecting search-ray and calls down the entire truth of divine Love to heal these malformations, to deliver mental, vital, physical love from their insufficiencies or their perversions and reveal to them their true abounding share of the intimacy and the oneness, the ascending ecstasy and the descending rapture.

All true Truth of love and of the works of love the psychic being accepts in their place: but its flame mounts always upward and it is eager to push the ascent from lesser to higher degrees of Truth, since it knows that only by the ascent to a highest Truth and the descent of that highest Truth can Love be delivered from the cross and placed upon the throne; for the cross is the sign of the Divine Descent barred and marred by the transversal line of a cosmic deformation which turns it into a stake of suffering and misfortune. Only by the ascent to the original Truth can the deformation be healed and all the works of love, as too all the works of knowledge and of life, be restored to a divine significance and become part of an integral spiritual existence.

CHAPTER VI. THE ASCENT OF THE SACRIFICE–2

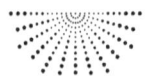

THE WORKS OF LOVE — THE WORKS OF LIFE

IT IS therefore through the sacrifice of love, works and knowledge with the psychic being as the leader and priest of the sacrifice that life itself can be transformed into its own true spiritual figure. If the sacrifice of knowledge rightly done is easily the largest and purest offering we can bring to the Highest, the sacrifice of love is not less demanded of us for our spiritual perfection; it is even more intense and rich in its singleness and can be made not less vast and pure. This pure wideness is brought into the intensity of the sacrifice of love when into all our activities there is poured the spirit and power of a divine infinite joy and the whole atmosphere of our life is suffused with an engrossing adoration of the One who is the All and the Highest. For then does the sacrifice of love attain its utter perfection when, offered to the divine All, it becomes integral, catholic and boundless, and when, uplifted to the Supreme, it ceases to be the weak, superficial and transient movement men call love and becomes a pure and grand and deep uniting Ananda.

Although it is a divine love for the supreme and universal Divine that must be the rule of our spiritual existence, this does not exclude altogether all forms of individual love or the ties that draw soul to soul in manifested existence. A psychic change is demanded, a divestiture of the masks of the Ignorance, a purification of the egoistic mental, vital and physical movements that prolong the old inferior consciousness; each movement of love, spiritualised, must depend no longer on mental preference, vital passion or physical craving, but on the recognition of soul by soul,—love restored to its fundamental spiritual and psychic essence with the mind, the vital, the physical as manifesting instruments and elements of that greater oneness.

In this change the individual love also is converted by a natural heightening into a divine love for the Divine Inhabitant immanent in a mind and soul and body occupied by the One in all creatures.

All love, indeed, that is adoration has a spiritual force behind it, and even when it is offered ignorantly and to a limited object, something of that splendour appears through the poverty of the rite and the smallness of its issues. For love that is worship is at once an aspiration and a preparation: it can bring even within its small limits in the Ignorance a glimpse of a still more or less blind and partial but surprising realisation; for there are moments when it is not we but the One who loves and is loved in us, and even a human passion can be uplifted and glorified by a slight glimpse of this infinite Love and Lover. It is for this reason that the worship of the god, the worship of the idol, the human magnet or ideal are not to be despised; for these are steps through which the human race moves towards that blissful passion and ecstasy of the Infinite which, even in limiting it, they yet represent for our imperfect vision when we have still to use the inferior steps Nature has hewn for our feet and admit the stages of our progress. Certain idolatries are indispensable for the development of our emotional being, nor will the man who knows be hasty at any time to shatter the image unless he can replace it in the heart of the worshipper by the Reality it figures. Moreover, they have this power because there is always something in them that is greater than their forms and, even when we reach the supreme worship, that abides and becomes a prolongation of it or a part of its catholic wholeness. Our knowledge is still imperfect in us, love incomplete if even when we know That which surpasses all forms and manifestations, we cannot still accept the Divine in creature and object, in man, in the kind, in the animal, in the tree, in the flower, in the work of our hands, in the Nature-Force which is then no longer to us the blind action of a material machinery but a face and power of the universal Shakti: for in these things too is the presence of the Eternal.

An ultimate inexpressible adoration offered by us to the Transcendent, to the Highest,[1] to the Ineffable, is yet no complete worship if it is not offered to him wherever he manifests or wherever even he hides his godhead—in man[2] and object and every creature. An Ignorance is there no doubt which imprisons the heart, distorts its feelings, obscures the significance of its offering; all partial worship, all religion which erects a mental or a physical idol is tempted to veil and protect the truth in it by a certain cloak of ignorance and easily loses the truth in its image. But the pride of exclusive knowledge is also a limitation and a barrier. For there is, concealed behind individual love, obscured by its ignorant human figure, a mystery which the mind cannot seize, the mystery of the body of the Divine, the secret of a mystic form of the Infinite which we can approach only through the ecstasy of the heart and the passion of the pure and sublimated sense, and its attraction which is the call of the divine Flute-player, the mastering compulsion of the AllBeautiful, can only be seized and seize us through an occult love and yearning which in the end makes one the Form and the Formless, and identifies Spirit and Matter. It is that which the spirit in Love is seeking here in the darkness of the Ignorance and it is that which it finds when individual human love is changed into the love of the Immanent Divine incarnate in the material universe.

As with individual, so with universal Love; all that widening of the self through sympathy, goodwill, universal benevolence and beneficence, love of mankind, love of creatures, the attraction of all the myriad forms and presences that surround us, by which mentally and emotionally man escapes from the first limits of his ego, has to be taken up into a unifying divine love for the universal Divine. Adoration fulfilled in love, love in Ananda,—the surpassing love, the self-wrapped ecstasy of transcendent delight in the Transcendent which awaits us at the end of the path of Devotion,—has for its wider result a universal love for all beings, the Ananda of all that is; we perceive behind every veil the Divine, spiritually embrace in all forms the All-Beautiful. A universal delight in his endless manifestation flows through us, taking in its surge every form and movement, but not bound or stationary in any and always reaching out to a greater and more perfect expression. This universal love is liberative and dynamic for transformation; for the discord of forms and appearances ceases to affect the heart that has felt the one Truth behind them all and understood their perfect significance. The impartial equality of soul of the selfless worker and knower is transformed by the magic touch of divine Love into an all-embracing ecstasy and million-bodied beatitude. All things become bodies and all movements the playings of the divine Beloved in his infinite house of pleasure. Even pain is changed and in their reaction and even in their essence things painful alter; the forms of pain fall away, there are created in their place the forms of Ananda.

This is in its essence the nature of the change of consciousness which turns existence itself into a glorified field of a Divine Love and Ananda. In its essence it begins for the seeker when he passes from the ordinary to the spiritual level and looks with a new heart of luminous vision and feeling on the world and self and others. It reaches its height when the spiritual becomes also the supramental level and then also it is possible not only to feel it in essence but realise it dynamically as a Power for the transformation of the whole inner life and the whole outer existence.

It is not altogether difficult for the mind to envisage, even though it may be difficult for the human will with its many earth-ties to accept, this transformation of the spirit and nature of love from the character of a mixed and limited human emotion to a supreme and all-embracing divine passion. It is when we come to the works of love that a certain perplexity is likely to intervene. It is possible, as in a certain high exaggeration of the path of knowledge, to cut here also the knot of the problem, escape the difficulty of uniting the spirit of love with the crudities of the world-action by avoiding it; it is open to us, withdrawing from outward life and action altogether, to live alone with our adoration of the Divine in the heart's silence. It is possible too to admit only those acts that are either in themselves an expression of love for the Divine, prayer, praise, symbolic acts of worship or subordinate activities that may be attached to these things and partake of their spirit, and to leave aside all else; the soul turns away to satisfy its inner longing in the absorbed or the God-centred life of the saint and devotee. It is possible, again, to open the doors of life more largely and to spend one's love of the Divine in acts of service to those around us and to the race; one can do the works of philanthropy, benevolence and beneficence, charity and succour to man and beast and every creature, transfigure them by a kind of spiritual passion, at least bring into their merely ethical appearance the greater power of a spiritual motive. This is indeed the solution most commonly favoured by the religious mind of today and we see it confidently advanced on all sides as the proper field of action of the God-seeker or of the man whose life is founded on divine love and knowledge. But the integral Yoga pushed towards a complete union of the Divine with the earth-life cannot stop short in this narrow province or limit this union within the lesser dimensions of an ethical rule of philanthropy and beneficence. All action must be made in it part of the God-life, our acts of knowledge, our acts of power and production and creation, our acts of joy and beauty and the soul's pleasure, our acts of will and endeavour and struggle and not our acts only of love and beneficent service. Its way to do these things will be not outward and mental, but inward and spiritual, and to that end it will bring into all activities, whatever they are, the spirit of divine love, the spirit of adoration and worship, the spirit of happiness in the Divine and in the beauty of the Divine so as to make all life a sacrifice of the works of the soul's love to the Divine, its cult of the Master of its existence.

It is possible so to turn life into an act of adoration to the Supreme by the spirit in one's works; for, says the Gita, "He who gives to me with a heart of adoration a leaf, a flower, a fruit or a cup of water, I take and enjoy that offering of his devotion"; and it is not only any dedicated external gift that can be so offered with love and devotion, but all our thoughts, all our feelings and sensations, all our outward activities and their forms and objects can be such gifts to the Eternal. It is true that the special act or form of action has its importance, even a great importance, but it is the spirit in the act that is the essential factor; the spirit of which it is the symbol or materialised expression gives it its whole value and justifying significance. Or it may be said that a complete act of divine love and worship has in it three parts that are the expressions of a single whole,—a practical worship of the Divine in the act, a symbol of worship in the form of the act expressing some vision and seeking or some relation with the Divine, an inner adoration and longing for oneness or feeling of oneness in the heart and soul and spirit. It is so that life can be changed into worship,—by putting behind it the spirit of a transcendent and universal love, the seeking of oneness, the sense of oneness; by making each act a symbol, an expression of Godward emotion or a relation with the Divine; by turning all we do into an act of worship, an act of the soul's communion, the mind's understanding, the life's obedience, the heart's surrender.

In any cult the symbol, the significant rite or expressive figure is not only a moving and enriching aesthetic element, but a physical means by which the human being begins to make outwardly definite the emotion and aspiration of his heart, to confirm it and to dynamise it. For if without a spiritual aspiration worship is meaningless and vain, yet the aspiration also without the act and the form is a disembodied and, for life, an incompletely effective power. It is unhappily the fate of all forms in human life to become crystallised, purely formal and therefore effete, and although form and cult preserve always their power for the man who can still enter into their meaning, the majority come to use the ceremony as a mechanical rite and the symbol as a lifeless sign, and because that kills the soul of religion, cult and form have in the end to be changed or thrown aside altogether. There are those even to whom all cult and form are for this reason suspect and offensive; but few can dispense with the support of outward symbols and, even, a certain divine element in human nature demands them always for the completeness of its spiritual satisfaction. Always the symbol is legitimate in so far as it is true, sincere, beautiful and delightful, and even one may say that a spiritual consciousness without any aesthetic or emotional content is not entirely or at any rate not integrally spiritual. In the spiritual life the basis of the act is a spiritual consciousness perennial and renovating, moved to express itself always in new forms or able to renew the truth of a form always by the flow of the spirit, and to so express itself and make every action a living symbol of some truth of the soul is the very nature of its creative vision and impulse. It is so that the spiritual seeker must deal with life and transmute its form and glorify it in its essence.

A supreme divine Love is a creative Power and, even though it can exist in itself silent and unchangeable, yet rejoices in external form and expression and is not condemned to be a speechless and bodiless godhead. It has even been said that creation itself was an act of love or at least the building up of a field in which Divine Love could devise its symbols and fulfil itself in act of mutuality and self-giving, and, if not the initial nature of creation, this may well be its ultimate object and motive. It does not so appear now because, even if a Divine Love is there in the world upholding all this evolution of creatures, yet the stuff of life and its action is made up of an egoistic formation, a division, a struggle of life and consciousness to exist and survive in an apparently indifferent, inclement or even hostile world of inanimate and inconscient Matter. In the confusion and obscurity of this struggle all are thrown against each other with a will in each to assert its own existence first and foremost and only secondarily to assert itself in others and very partially for others; for even man's altruism remains essentially egoistic and must be so till the soul finds the secret of the divine Oneness. It is to discover that at its supreme source, to bring it from within and to radiate it out up to the extreme confines of life that is turned the effort of the Yoga. All action, all creation must be turned into a form, a symbol of the cult, the adoration, the sacrifice; it must carry something that makes it bear in it the stamp of a dedication, a reception and translation of the Divine Consciousness, a service of the Beloved, a self-giving, a surrender. This has to be done wherever possible in the outward body and form of the act; it must be done always in its inward emotion and an intensity that shows it to be an outflow from the soul towards the Eternal.

In itself the adoration in the act is a great and complete and powerful sacrifice that tends by its self-multiplication to reach the discovery of the One and make the radiation of the Divine possible. For devotion by its embodiment in acts not only makes its own way broad and full and dynamic, but brings at once into the harder way of works in the world the divinely passionate element of joy and love which is often absent in its beginning when it is only the austere spiritual Will that follows in a struggling uplifting tension the steep ascent, and the heart is still asleep or bound to silence. If the spirit of divine love can enter, the hardness of the way diminishes, the tension is lightened, there is a sweetness and joy even in the core of difficulty and struggle. The indispensable surrender of all our will and works and activities to the Supreme is indeed only perfect and perfectly effective when it is a surrender of love. All life turned into this cult, all actions done in the love of the Divine and in the love of the world and its creatures seen and felt as the Divine manifested in many disguises become by that very fact part of an integral Yoga.

It is the inner offering of the heart's adoration, the soul of it in the symbol, the spirit of it in the act, that is the very life of the sacrifice. If this offering is to be complete and universal, then a turning of all our emotions to the Divine is imperative. This is the intensest way of purification for the human heart, more powerful than any ethical or aesthetic catharsis could ever be by its half-power and superficial pressure. A psychic fire within must be lit into which all is thrown with the Divine Name upon it. In that fire all the emotions are compelled to cast off their grosser elements and those that are undivine perversions are burned away and the others discard their insufficiencies, till a spirit of largest love and a stainless divine delight arises out of the flame and smoke and frankincense. It is the divine love which so emerges that, extended in inward feeling to the Divine in man and all creatures in an active universal equality, will be more potent for the perfectibility of life and a more real instrument than the ineffective mental ideal of brotherhood can ever be. It is this poured out into acts that could alone create a harmony in the world and a true unity between all its creatures; all else strives in vain towards that end so long as Divine Love has not disclosed itself as the heart of the delivered manifestation in terrestrial Nature.

It is here that the emergence of the secret psychic being in us as the leader of the sacrifice is of the utmost importance; for this inmost being alone can bring with it the full power of the spirit in the act, the soul in the symbol. It alone can assure, even while the spiritual consciousness is incomplete, the perennial freshness and sincerity and beauty of the symbol and prevent it from becoming a dead form or a corrupted and corrupting magic; it alone can preserve for the act its power with its significance. All the other members of our being, mind, life-force, physical or body consciousness, are too much under the control of the Ignorance to be a sure instrumentation and much less can they be a guide or the source of an unerring impulse. Always the greater part of the motive and action of these powers clings to the old law, the deceiving tablets, the cherished inferior movements of Nature and they meet with reluctance, alarm or revolt or obstructing inertia the voices and the forces that call and impel us to exceed and transform ourselves into a greater being and a wider Nature. In their major part the response is either a resistance or a qualified or temporising acquiescence; for even if they follow the call, they yet tend—when not consciously, then by automatic habit—to bring into the spiritual action their own natural disabilities and errors. At every moment they are moved to take egoistic advantage of the psychic and spiritual influences and can be detected using the power, joy or light these bring into us for a lower life-motive. Afterwards too, even when the seeker has opened to the Divine Love transcendental, universal or immanent, yet if he tries to pour it into life, he meets the power of obscuration and perversion of these lower Nature-forces. Always they draw away towards pitfalls, pour into that higher intensity their diminishing elements, seek to capture the descending Power for themselves and their interests and degrade it into an aggrandised mental, vital or physical instrumentation for desire and ego. Instead of a Divine Love creator of a new heaven and a new earth of Truth and Light, they would hold it here prisoner as a tremendous sanction and glorifying force of sublimation to gild the mud of the old earth and colour with its rose and sapphire the old turbid unreal skies of sentimentalising vital imagination and mental idealised chimera. If that falsification is permitted, the higher Light and Power and Bliss withdraw, there is a fall back to a lower status; or else the realisation remains tied to an insecure half-way and mixture or is covered and even submerged by an inferior exaltation that is not the true Ananda. It is for this reason that Divine Love which is at the heart of all creation and the most powerful of all redeeming and creative forces has yet been the least frontally present in earthly life, the least successfully redemptive, the least creative. Human nature has been unable to bear it in its purity for the very reason that it is the most powerful, pure, rare and intense of all the divine energies; what little could be seized has been corrupted at once into a vital pietistic ardour, a defenceless religious or ethical sentimentalism, a sensuous or even sensual erotic mysticism of the roseate coloured mind or passionately turbid life-impulse and with these simulations compensated its inability to house the Mystic Flame that could rebuild the world with its tongues of sacrifice. It is only the inmost psychic being unveiled and emerging in its full power that can lead the pilgrim sacrifice unscathed through these ambushes and pitfalls; at each moment it catches, exposes, repels the mind's and the life's falsehoods, seizes hold on the truth of the Divine Love and Ananda and separates it from the excitement of the mind's ardours and the blind enthusiasms of the misleading life-force. But all things that are true at their core in mind and life and the physical being it extricates and takes with it in the journey till they stand on the heights, new in spirit and sublime in figure.

And yet even the leading of the inmost psychic being is not found sufficient until it has succeeded in raising itself out of this mass of inferior Nature to the highest spiritual levels and the divine spark and flame descended here have rejoined themselves to their original fiery Ether. For there is there no longer a spiritual consciousness still imperfect and half lost to itself in the thick sheaths of human mind, life and body, but the full spiritual consciousness in its purity, freedom and intense wideness. There, as it is the eternal Knower that becomes the Knower in us and mover and user of all knowledge, so it is the eternal All-Blissful who is the Adored attracting to himself the eternal divine portion of his being and joy that has gone out into the play of the universe, the infinite Lover pouring himself out in the multiplicity of his own manifested selves in a happy Oneness. All Beauty in the world is there the beauty of the Beloved, and all forms of beauty have to stand under the light of that eternal Beauty and submit themselves to the sublimating and transfiguring power of the unveiled Divine Perfection. All Bliss and Joy are there of the All-Blissful, and all inferior forms of enjoyment, happiness or pleasure are subjected to the shock of the intensity of its floods or currents and either they are broken to pieces as inadequate things under its convicting stress or compelled to transmute themselves into the forms of the Divine Ananda. Thus for the individual consciousness a Force is manifested which can deal sovereignly in it with the diminutions and degradations of the values of the Ignorance. At last it begins to be possible to bring down into life the immense reality and intense concreteness of the love and joy that are of the Eternal. Or at any rate it will be possible for our spiritual consciousness to raise itself out of mind into the supramental Light and Force and Vastness; there in the light and potency of the supramental Gnosis are the splendour and joy of a power of divine self-expression and self-organisation which could rescue and re-create even the world of the Ignorance into a figure of the Truth of the Spirit.

There in the supramental Gnosis is the fulfilment, the culminating height, the all-embracing extent of the inner adoration, the profound and integral union, the flaming wings of Love upbearing the power and joy of a supreme Knowledge. For supramental Love brings an active ecstasy that surpasses the void passive peace and stillness which is the heaven of the liberated Mind and does not betray the deeper greater calm which is the beginning of the supramental silence. The unity of a love which is able to include in itself all differences without being diminished or abrogated by their present limitations and apparent dissonances is raised to its full potentiality on the supramental level. For there an intense oneness with all creatures founded on a profound oneness of the soul with the Divine can harmonise with a play of relations that only makes the oneness more perfect and absolute. The power of Love supramentalised can take hold of all living relations without hesitation or danger and turn them Godwards delivered from their crude, mixed and petty human settings and sublimated into the happy material of a divine life. For it is the very nature of the supramental experience that it can perpetuate the play of difference without forfeiting or in the least diminishing either the divine union or the infinite oneness. For a supramentalised consciousness it would be utterly possible to embrace all contacts with men and the world in a purified flame-force and with a transfigured significance, because the soul would then perceive always as the object of all emotion and all seeking for love or beauty the One Eternal and could spiritually use a wide and liberated life-urge to meet and join with that One Divine in all things and all creatures.

∼

Into the third and last category of the works of sacrifice can be gathered all that is directly proper to the Yoga of works; for here is its direct field of effectuation and major province. It covers the entire range of life's more visible activities; under it fall the multiform energies of the Will-to-Life throwing itself outward to make the most of material existence. It is here that an ascetic or other-worldly spirituality feels an insurmountable denial of the Truth which it seeks after and is compelled to turn away from terrestrial existence, rejecting it as for ever the dark playground of an incurable Ignorance. Yet it is precisely these activities that are claimed for a spiritual conquest and divine transformation by the integral Yoga. Abandoned altogether by the more ascetic disciplines, accepted by others only as a field of temporary ordeal or a momentary, superficial and ambiguous play of the concealed spirit, this existence is fully embraced and welcomed by the integral seeker as a field of fulfilment, a field for divine works, a field of the total self-discovery of the concealed and indwelling spirit. A discovery of the Divinity in oneself is his first object, but a total discovery too of the Divinity in the world behind the apparent denial offered by its scheme and figures and, last, a total discovery of the dynamism of some transcendent Eternal; for by its descent this world and self will be empowered to break their disguising envelopes and become divine in revealing form and manifesting process as they now are secretly in their hidden essence.

This object of the integral Yoga must be accepted wholly by those who follow it, but the acceptance must not be in ignorance of the immense stumbling-blocks that lie in the way of the achievement; on the contrary we must be fully aware of the compelling cause of the refusal of so many other disciplines to regard even its possibility, much less its imperative character, as the true meaning of terrestrial existence. For here in the works of life in the earth-nature is the very heart of the difficulty that has driven Philosophy to its heights of aloofness and turned away even the eager eye of Religion from the malady of birth in a mortal body to a distant Paradise or a silent peace of Nirvana. A way of pure Knowledge is comparatively straightforward and easy to the tread of the seeker in spite of our mental limitations and the pitfalls of the Ignorance; a way of pure Love, although it has its stumbling-blocks and its sufferings and trials, can in comparison be as easy as the winging of a bird through the free azure. For Knowledge and Love are pure in their essence and become mixed and embarrassed, corrupted and degraded only when they enter into the ambiguous movement of the life-forces and are seized by them for the outward life's crude movements and obstinately inferior motives. Alone of the three powers Life or at least a certain predominant Will-in-Life has the appearance of something impure, accursed or fallen in its very essence. At its contact, wrapped in its dull sheaths or caught in its iridescent quagmires, the divinities themselves become common and muddy and hardly escape from being dragged downwards into its perversions and disastrously assimilated to the demon and the Asura. A principle of dark and dull inertia is at its base; all are tied down by the body and its needs and desires to a trivial mind, petty desires and emotions, an insignificant repetition of small worthless functionings, needs, cares, occupations, pains, pleasures that lead to nothing beyond themselves and bear the stamp of an ignorance that knows not its own why and whither. This physical mind of inertia believes in no divinity other than its own small earth-gods; it aspires perhaps to a greater comfort, order, pleasure, but asks for no uplifting and no spiritual deliverance. At the centre we meet a stronger Will of life with a greater gusto, but it is a blinded Daemon, a perverted spirit and exults in the very elements that make of life a striving turmoil and an unhappy imbroglio. It is a soul of human or Titanic desire clinging to the garish colour, disordered poetry, violent tragedy or stirring melodrama of this mixed flux of good and evil, joy and sorrow, light and darkness, heady rapture and bitter torture. It loves these things and would have more and more of them or, even when it suffers and cries out against them, can accept or joy in nothing else; it hates and revolts against higher things and in its fury would trample, tear or crucify any diviner Power that has the presumption to offer to make life pure, luminous and happy and snatch from its lips the fiery brew of that exciting mixture. Another Will-in-Life there is that is ready to follow the ameliorating ideal Mind and is allured by its offer to extract some harmony, beauty, light, nobler order out of life, but this is a smaller part of the vital nature and can be easily overpowered by its more violent or darker duller yoke-comrades; nor does it readily lend itself to a call higher than that of the Mind unless that call defeats itself, as Religion usually does, by lowering its demand to conditions more intelligible to our obscure vital nature. All these forces the spiritual seeker grows aware of in himself and finds all around him and has to struggle and combat incessantly to be rid of their grip and dislodge the long-entrenched mastery they have exercised over his own being as over the environing human existence. The difficulty is great; for their hold is so strong, so apparently invincible that it justifies the disdainful dictum which compares human nature to a dog's tail,—for, straighten it never so much by force of ethics, religion, reason or any other redemptive effort, it returns in the end always to the crooked curl of Nature. And so great is the vim, the clutch of that more agitated Life-Will, so immense the peril of its passions and errors, so subtly insistent or persistently invasive, so obstinate up to the very gates of Heaven the fury of its attack or the tedious obstruction of its obstacles that even the saint and the Yogin cannot be sure of their liberated purity or their trained self-mastery against its intrigue or its violence. All labour to straighten out this native crookedness strikes the struggling will as a futility; a flight, a withdrawal to happy Heaven or peaceful dissolution easily finds credit as the only wisdom and to find a way not to be born again gets established as the only remedy for the dull bondage or the poor shoddy delirium or the blinded and precarious happiness and achievement of earthly existence.

A remedy yet there should be and is, a way of redress and a chance of transformation for this troubled vital nature; but for that the cause of deviation must be found and remedied at the heart of Life itself and in its very principle, since Life too is a power of the Divine and not a creation of some malignant Chance or dark Titanic impulse, however obscure or perverted may be its actual appearance. In Life itself there is the seed of its own salvation, it is from the Life-Energy that we must get our leverage; for though there is a saving light in Knowledge, a redeeming and transforming force in Love, these cannot be effective here unless they secure the consent of Life and can use the instrumentation of some delivered energy at its centre for a sublimation of the erring human into a divine Life-Force. It is not possible to cut the difficulty by a splitting up of the works of sacrifice; we cannot escape it by deciding that we shall do only the works of Love and Knowledge and leave aside the works of will and power, possession and acquisition, production and fruitful expense of capacity, battle and victory and mastery, striking away from us the larger part of life because it seems to be made of the very stuff of desire and ego and therefore doomed to be a field of disharmony and mere conflict and disorder. For the division cannot really be made; or, if attempted, it must fail in its essential purpose, since it would isolate us from the total energies of the World-Power and sterilise an important part of integral Nature, just the one force in it that is a necessary instrument in any world-creative purpose. The Life-Force is an indispensable intermediary, the effectuating element in Nature here; mind needs its alliance if the works of mind are not to remain shining inner formations without a body; the spirit needs it to give an outer force and form to its manifested possibilities and arrive at a complete self-expression incarnated in Matter. If Life refuses the aid of its intermediary energy to the spirit's other workings or is itself refused, they are likely to be reduced for all the effect they can have here to a static seclusion or a golden impotence; or if anything is done, it will be a partial irradiation of our action more subjective than objective, modifying existence perhaps, but without force to change it. Yet if Life brings its forces to the spirit but unregenerate, a worse result may follow since it is likely to reduce the spiritual action of Love or Knowledge to diminished and corrupted motions or make them accomplices of its own inferior or perverse workings. Life is indispensable to the completeness of the creative spiritual realisation, but life released, transformed, uplifted, not the ordinary mentalised human-animal life, nor the demoniac or Titanic, nor even the divine and the undivine mixed together. Whatever may be done by other world-shunning or heaven-seeking disciplines, this is the difficult but unavoidable task of the integral Yoga; it cannot afford to leave unsolved the problem of the outward works of Life, it must find in them their native Divinity and ally it firmly and for ever to the divinities of Love and Knowledge.

It is no solution either to postpone dealing with the works of Life till Love and Knowledge have been evolved to a point at which they can sovereignly and with safety lay hold on the Life-Force to regenerate it; for we have seen that they have to rise to immense heights before they can be secure from the vital perversion which hampers or hamstrings their power to deliver. If once our consciousness could reach the heights of a supramental Nature, then indeed these disabilities would disappear. But here there is the dilemma that it is impossible to reach the supramental heights with the burden of an unregenerated LifeForce on our shoulders and equally impossible to regenerate radically the Will-in-Life without bringing down the infallible light and unconquerable power that belong to the spiritual and supramental levels. The Supramental Consciousness is not only a Knowledge, a Bliss, an intimate Love and Oneness, it is also a Will, a principle of Power and Force, and it cannot descend till the element of Will, of Power, of Force in this manifested Nature is sufficiently developed and sublimated to receive and bear it. But Will, Power, Force are the native substance of the Life-Energy, and herein lies the justification for the refusal of Life to acknowledge the supremacy of Knowledge and Love alone,—for its push towards the satisfaction of something far more unreflecting, headstrong and dangerous that can yet venture too in its own bold and ardent way towards the Divine and Absolute. Love and Wisdom are not the only aspects of the Divine, there is also its aspect of Power. As the mind gropes for Knowledge, as the heart feels out for Love, so the life-force, however fumblingly or trepidantly, stumbles in search of Power and the control given by Power. It is a mistake of the ethical or religious mind to condemn Power as in itself a thing not to be accepted or sought after because naturally corrupting and evil; in spite of its apparent justification by a majority of instances, this is at its core a blind and irrational prejudice. However corrupted and misused, as Love and Knowledge too are corrupted and misused, Power is divine and put here for a divine use. Shakti, Will, Power is the driver of the worlds and, whether it be Knowledge-Force or Love-Force or Life-Force or Action-Force or Body-Force, is always spiritual in its origin and divine in its native character. It is the use of it made in the Ignorance by brute, man or Titan that has to be cast aside and replaced by its greater natural—even if to us supernormal—action led by the Light of an inner consciousness which is in tune with the Infinite and the Eternal. The integral Yoga cannot reject the works of Life and be satisfied with an inward experience only; it has to go inward in order to change the outward, making the Life-Force a part and a working of a Yoga-Energy which is in touch with the Divine and divine in its guidance.

All the difficulty in dealing spiritually with the works of Life arises because the Will-in-Life for its purposes in the Ignorance has created a false soul of desire and substituted it for that spark of the Divine which is the true psyche. All or most of the works of life are at present or seem to be actuated and vitiated by this soul of desire; even those that are ethical or religious, even those that wear the guise of altruism, philanthropy, self-sacrifice, self-denial, are shot through and through with the threads of its making. This soul of desire is a separative soul of ego and all its instincts are for a separative self-affirmation; it pushes always, openly or under more or less shining masks, for its own growth, for possession, for enjoyment, for conquest and empire. If the curse of disquiet and disharmony and perversion is to be lifted from Life, the true soul, the psychic being, must be given its leading place and there must be a dissolution of the false soul of desire and ego. But this does not mean that life itself must be coerced and denied its native line of fulfilment; for behind this outer life soul of desire there is in us an inner and true vital being which has not to be dissolved but brought out into prominence and released to its true working as a power of the Divine Nature. The prominence of this true vital being under the lead of the true inmost soul within us is the condition for the divine fulfilment of the objects of the Life-Force. Those objects will even remain the same in essence, but transformed in their inner motive and outer character. The Divine Life-Power too will be a will for growth, a force of self-affirmation, but affirmation of the Divine within us, not of the little temporary personality on the surface,—growth into the true divine Individual, the central being, the secret imperishable Person who can emerge only by the subordination and disappearance of the ego. This is life's true object: growth, but a growth of the spirit in Nature, affirming and developing itself in mind, life and body; possession, but a possession by the Divine of the Divine in all things, and not of things for their own sake by the desire of the ego; enjoyment, but an enjoyment of the divine Ananda in the universe; battle and conquest and empire in the shape of a victorious conflict with the Powers of Darkness, an entire spiritual self-rule and mastery over inward and outward Nature, a conquest by Knowledge, Love and Divine Will over the domains of the Ignorance.

These are the conditions and these must be the aims of the divine effectuation of the works of Life and their progressive transformation which is the third element of the triple sacrifice. It is not a rationalisation but a supramentalisation, not a moralising but a spiritualising of life that is the object of the Yoga. It is not a handling of externals or superficial psychological motives that is its main purpose, but a refounding of life and its action on their hidden divine element; for only such a refounding of life can bring about its direct government by the secret Divine Power above us and its transfiguration into a manifest expression of the Divinity, not as now a disguise and a disfiguring mask of the eternal Actor. It is a spiritual essential change of consciousness, not the surface manipulation which is the method of Mind and Reason, that can alone make Life other than it now is and rescue it out of its present distressed and ambiguous figure.

It is then by a transformation of life in its very principle, not by an external manipulation of its phenomena, that the integral Yoga proposes to change it from a troubled and ignorant into a luminous and harmonious movement of Nature. There are three conditions which are indispensable for the achievement of this central inner revolution and new formation; none of them is altogether sufficient in itself, but by their united threefold power the uplifting can be done, the conversion made and completely made. For, first, life as it is is a movement of desire and it has built in us as its centre a desire-soul which refers to itself all the motions of life and puts in them its own troubled hue and pain of an ignorant, half-lit, baffled endeavour: for a divine living, desire must be abolished and replaced by a purer and firmer motivepower, the tormented soul of desire dissolved and in its stead there must emerge the calm, strength, happiness of a true vital being now concealed within us. Next, life as it is is driven or led partly by the impulse of the life-force, partly by a mind which is mostly a servant and abettor of the ignorant life-impulse, but in part also its uneasy and not too luminous or competent guide and mentor; for a divine life the mind and the life-impulse must cease to be anything but instruments and the inmost psychic being must take their place as the leader on the path and the indicator of a divine guidance. Last, life as it is is turned towards the satisfaction of the separative ego; ego must disappear and be replaced by the true spiritual person, the central being, and life itself must be turned towards the fulfilment of the Divine in terrestrial existence; it must feel a Divine Force awaking within it and become an obedient instrumentation of its purpose.

There is nothing that is not ancient and familiar in the first of these three transforming inner movements; for it has always been one of the principal objects of spiritual discipline. It has been best formulated in the already expressed doctrine of the Gita by which a complete renouncement of desire for the fruits as the motive of action, a complete annulment of desire itself, the complete achievement of a perfect equality are put forward as the normal status of a spiritual being. A perfect spiritual equality is the one true and infallible sign of the cessation of desire,—to be equal-souled to all things, unmoved by joy and sorrow, the pleasant and the unpleasant, success or failure, to look with an equal eye on high and low, friend and enemy, the virtuous and the sinner, to see in all beings the manifold manifestation of the One and in all things the multitudinous play or the slow masked evolution of the embodied Spirit. It is not a mental quiet, aloofness, indifference, not an inert vital quiescence, not a passivity of the physical consciousness consenting to no movement or to any movement that is the condition aimed at, though these things are sometimes mistaken for this spiritual condition, but a wide comprehensive unmoved universality such as that of the Witness Spirit behind Nature. For all here seems to be a mobile half-ordered half-confused organisation of forces, but behind them one can feel a supporting peace, silence, wideness, not inert but calm, not impotent but potentially omnipotent with a concentrated, stable, immobile energy in it capable of bearing all the motions of the universe. This Presence behind is equal-souled to all things: the energy it holds in it can be unloosed for any action, but no action will be chosen by any desire in the Witness Spirit; a Truth acts which is beyond and greater than the action itself or its apparent forms and impulses, beyond and greater than mind or life-force or body, although it may take for the immediate purpose a mental, a vital or a physical appearance. It is when there is this death of desire and this calm equal wideness in the consciousness everywhere, that the true vital being within us comes out from the veil and reveals its own calm, intense and potent presence. For such is the true nature of the vital being, *prāṇamaya puruṣa*; it is a projection of the Divine Purusha into life,—tranquil, strong, luminous, many-energied, obedient to the Divine Will, egoless, yet or rather therefore capable of all action, achievement, highest or largest enterprise. The true Life-Force too reveals itself as no longer this troubled harassed divided striving surface energy, but a great and radiant Divine Power, full of peace and strength and bliss, a wide-wayed Angel of Life with its wings of Might enfolding the universe.

And yet this transformation into a large strength and equality is insufficient; for if it opens to us the instrumentation of a Divine Life, it does not provide its government and initiative. It is here that the presence of the released psychic being intervenes; it does not give the supreme government and direction,—for that is not its function,—but it supplies during the transition from ignorance to a divine Knowledge a progressive guidance for the inner and outer life and action; it indicates at each moment the method, the way, the steps that will lead to that fulfilled spiritual condition in which a supreme dynamic initiative will be always there directing the activities of a divinised Life-Force.

The light it sheds illuminates the other parts of the nature which, for want of any better guidance than their own confused and groping powers, have been wandering in the rounds of the Ignorance; it gives to mind the intrinsic feeling of the thoughts and perceptions, to life the infallible sense of the movements that are misled or misleading and those that are well-inspired; something like a quiet oracle from within discloses the causes of our stumblings, warns in time against their repetition, extracts from experience and intuition the law, not rigid but plastic, of a just direction for our acts, a right stepping, an accurate impulse. A will is created that becomes more in consonance with evolving Truth rather than with the circling and dilatory mazes of a seeking Error. A determined orientation towards the greater Light to be, a soul-instinct, a psychic tact and insight into the true substance, motion and intention of things, coming always nearer and nearer to a spiritual vision, to a knowledge by inner contact, inner sight and even identity, begin to replace the superficial keenness of mental judgment and the eager graspings of the life-force. The works of Life right themselves, escape from confusion, substitute for the artificial or legal order imposed by the intellect and for the arbitrary rule of desire the guidance of the soul's inner insight, enter into the profound paths of the Spirit. Above all, the psychic being imposes on life the law of the sacrifice of all its works as an offering to the Divine and the Eternal. Life becomes a call to that which is beyond Life; its every smallest act enlarges with the sense of the Infinite.

As an inner equality increases and with it the sense of the true vital being waiting for the greater direction it has to serve, as the psychic call too increases in all the members of our nature, That to which the call is addressed begins to reveal itself, descends to take possession of the life and its energies and fills them with the height, intimacy, vastness of its presence and its purpose. In many, if not most, it manifests something of itself even before the equality and the open psychic urge or guidance are there. A call of the veiled psychic element oppressed by the mass of the outer ignorance and crying for deliverance, a stress of eager meditation and seeking for knowledge, a longing of the heart, a passionate will ignorant yet but sincere may break the lid that shuts off that Higher from this Lower Nature and open the floodgates. A little of the Divine Person may reveal itself or some Light, Power, Bliss, Love out of the Infinite. This may be a momentary revelation, a flash or a brief-lived gleam that soon withdraws and waits for the preparation of the nature; but also it may repeat itself, grow, endure. A long and large and comprehensive working will then have begun, sometimes luminous or intense, sometimes slow and obscure. A Divine Power comes in front at times and leads and compels or instructs and enlightens; at others it withdraws into the background and seems to leave the being to its own resources. All that is ignorant, obscure, perverted or simply imperfect and inferior in the being is raised up, perhaps brought to its acme, dealt with, corrected, exhausted, shown its own disastrous results, compelled to call for its own cessation or transformation or expelled as worthless or incorrigible from the nature. This cannot be a smooth and even process; alternations there are of day and night, illumination and darkness, calm and construction or battle and upheaval, the presence of the growing Divine Consciousness and its absence, heights of hope and abysses of despair, the clasp of the Beloved and the anguish of its absence, the overwhelming invasion, the compelling deceit, the fierce opposition, the disabling mockery of hostile Powers or the help and comfort and communion of the Gods and the Divine Messengers. A great and long revolution and churning of the ocean of Life with strong emergences of its nectar and its poison is enforced till all is ready and the increasing Descent finds a being, a nature prepared and conditioned for its complete rule and its all-encompassing presence. But if the equality and the psychic light and will are already there, then this process, though it cannot be dispensed with, can still be much lightened and facilitated: it will be rid of its worst dangers; and inner calm, happiness, confidence will support the steps through all the difficulties and trials of the transformation and the growing Force profiting by the full assent of the nature will rapidly diminish and eliminate the power of the opposing forces. A sure guidance and protection will be present throughout, sometimes standing in front, sometimes working behind the veil, and the power of the end will be already there even in the beginning and in the long middle stages of the great endeavour. For at all times the seeker will be aware of the Divine Guide and Protector or the working of the supreme Mother-Force; he will know that all is done for the best, the progress assured, the victory inevitable. In either case the process is the same and unavoidable, a taking up of the whole nature, of the whole life, of the internal and of the external, to reveal and handle and transform its forces and their movements under the pressure of a diviner Life from above, until all here has been possessed by greater spiritual powers and made an instrumentation of a spiritual action and a divine purpose.

In this process and at an early stage of it it becomes evident that what we know of ourselves, our present conscious existence, is only a representative formation, a superficial activity, a changing external result of a vast mass of concealed existence. Our visible life and the actions of that life are no more than a series of significant expressions, but that which it tries to express is not on the surface; our existence is something much larger than this apparent frontal being which we suppose ourselves to be and which we offer to the world around us. This frontal and external being is a confused amalgam of mind-formations, life-movements, physical functionings of which even an exhaustive analysis into its component parts and machinery fails to reveal the whole secret. It is only when we go behind, below, above into the hidden stretches of our being that we can know it; the most thorough and acute surface scrutiny and manipulation cannot give us the true understanding or the completely effective control of our life, its purposes, its activities; that inability indeed is the cause of the failure of reason, morality and every other surface action to control and deliver and perfect the life of the human race. For below even our most obscure physical consciousness is a subconscious being in which as in a covering and supporting soil are all manner of hidden seeds that sprout up, unaccountably to us, on our surface and into which we are constantly throwing fresh seeds that prolong our past and will influence our future,— a subconscious being, obscure, small in its motions, capriciously and almost fantastically subrational, but of an immense potency for the earth-life. Again behind our mind, our life, our conscious physical there is a larger subliminal consciousness,—there are inner mental, inner vital, inner more subtle physical reaches supported by an inmost psychic existence which is the animating soul of all the rest; and in these hidden reaches too lie a mass of numerous pre-existent personalities which supply the material, the motive-forces, the impulsions of our developing surface existence. For in each one of us here there may be one central person, but also a multitude of subordinate personalities created by the past history of its manifestation or by expressions of it on these inner planes which support its present play in this external material cosmos. And while on our surface we are cut off from all around us except through an exterior mind and sense contact which delivers but little of us to our world or of our world to us, in these inner reaches the barrier between us and the rest of existence is thin and easily broken; there we can feel at once —not merely infer from their results, but feel directly—the action of the secret world-forces, mind-forces, life-forces, subtle physical forces that constitute universal and individual existence; we shall even be able, if we will but train ourselves to it, to lay our hands on these world-forces that throw themselves on us or surround us and more and more to control or at least strongly modify their action on us and others, their formations, their very movements. Yet again, above our human mind are still greater reaches superconscient to it and from there secretly descend influences, powers, touches which are the original determinants of things here and, if they were called down in their fullness, could altogether alter the whole make and economy of life in the material universe. It is all this latent experience and knowledge that the Divine Force working upon us by our opening to it in the integral Yoga, progressively reveals to us, uses and works out the consequences as means and steps towards a transformation of our whole being and nature. Our life is thenceforth no longer a little rolling wave on the surface, but interpenetrant if not coincident with the cosmic life. Our spirit, our self rises not only into an inner identity with some wide cosmic Self but into some contact with that which is beyond, though aware of and dominant over the action of the universe.

It is thus by an integralisation of our divided being that the Divine Shakti in the Yoga will proceed to its object; for liberation, perfection, mastery are dependent on this integralisation, since the little wave on the surface cannot control its own movement, much less have any true control over the vast life around it. The Shakti, the power of the Infinite and the Eternal descends within us, works, breaks up our present psychological formations, shatters every wall, widens, liberates, presents us with always newer and greater powers of vision, ideation, perception and newer and greater life-motives, enlarges and newmodels increasingly the soul and its instruments, confronts us with every imperfection in order to convict and destroy it, opens to a greater perfection, does in a brief period the work of many lives or ages so that new births and new vistas open constantly within us. Expansive in her action, she frees the consciousness from confinement in the body; it can go out in trance or sleep or even waking and enter into worlds or other regions of this world and act there or carry back its experience. It spreads out, feeling the body only as a small part of itself, and begins to contain what before contained it; it achieves the cosmic consciousness and extends itself to be commensurate with the universe. It begins to know inwardly and directly and not merely by external observation and contact the forces at play in the world, feels their movement, distinguishes their functioning and can operate immediately upon them as the scientist operates upon physical forces, accept their action and results in our mind, life, body or reject them or modify, change, reshape, create immense new powers and movements in place of the old small functionings of the nature. We begin to perceive the working of the forces of universal Mind and to know how our thoughts are created by that working, separate from within the truth and falsehood of our perceptions, enlarge their field, extend and illumine their significance, become master of our own minds and active to shape the movements of Mind in the world around us. We begin to perceive the flow and surge of the universal life-forces, detect the origin and law of our feelings, emotions, sensations, passions, are free to accept, reject, new-create, open to wider, rise to higher planes of Life-Power. We begin to perceive too the key to the enigma of Matter, follow the interplay of Mind and Life and Consciousness upon it, discover more and more its instrumental and resultant function and detect ultimately the last secret of Matter as a form not merely of Energy but of involved and arrested or unstably fixed and restricted consciousness and begin to see too the possibility of its liberation and plasticity of response to higher Powers, its possibilities for the conscious and no longer the more than half-inconscient incarnation and self-expression of the Spirit. All this and more becomes more and more possible as the working of the Divine Shakti increases in us and, against much resistance or labour to respond of our obscure consciousness, through much struggle and movement of progress and regression and renewed progress necessitated by the work of intensive transformation of a half-inconscient into a conscious substance, moves to a greater purity, truth, height, range. All depends on the psychic awakening in us, the completeness of our response to her and our growing surrender.

But all this can only constitute a greater inner life with a greater possibility of the outer action and is a transitional achievement; the full transformation can come only by the ascent of the sacrifice to its farthest heights and its action upon life with the power and light and beatitude of the divine supramental Gnosis. For then alone all the forces that are divided and express themselves imperfectly in life and its works are raised to their original unity, harmony, single truth, authentic absoluteness and entire significance. There Knowledge and Will are one, Love and Force a single movement; the opposites that afflict us here are resolved into their reconciled unity: good develops its absolute and evil divesting itself of its error returns to the good that was behind it; sin and virtue vanish in a divine purity and an infallible truth-movement; the dubious evanescence of pleasure disappears in a Bliss that is the play of an eternal and happy spiritual certitude, and pain in perishing discovers the touch of an Ananda which was betrayed by some dark perversion and incapacity of the will of the Inconscient to receive it. These things, to the Mind an imagination or a mystery, become evident and capable of experience as the consciousness rises out of limited embodied Matter-mind to the freedom and fullness of the higher and higher ranges of the super-intelligence; but they can become entirely true and normal only when the supramental becomes the law of the nature.

It is therefore on the accomplishment of this ascent and on the possibility of a full dynamism from these highest levels descending into earth-consciousness that is dependent the justification of Life, its salvation, its transformation into a Divine Life in a transfigured terrestrial Nature.

~

The nature of the integral Yoga so conceived, so conditioned, progressing by these spiritual means, turning upon this integral transformation of the nature, determines of itself its answer to the question of the ordinary activities of life and their place in the Yoga.

There is not and cannot be here any ascetic or contemplative or mystic abandonment of works and life altogether, any gospel of an absorbed meditation and inactivity, any cutting away or condemnation of the Life-Force and its activities, any rejection of the manifestation in the earth-nature. It may be necessary for the seeker at any period to withdraw into himself, to remain plunged in his inner being, to shut out from him the noise and turmoil of the life of the Ignorance until a certain inner change has been accomplished or something achieved without which a further effective action on life has become difficult or impossible. But this can only be a period or an episode, a temporary necessity or a preparatory spiritual manoeuvre; it cannot be the rule of his Yoga or its principle.

A splitting up of the activities of human existence on a religious or an ethical basis or both together, a restriction to the works of worship only or to the works of philanthropy and beneficence only would be contrary to the spirit of the integral Yoga. Any merely mental rule or merely mental acceptance or repudiation is alien to the purpose and method of its discipline. All must be taken to a spiritual height and placed upon a spiritual basis; the presence of an inner spiritual change and an outer transformation must be enforced upon the whole of life and not merely on a part of life; all must be accepted that is helpful towards this change or admits it, all must be rejected that is incapable or inapt or refuses to submit itself to the transforming movement. There must be no attachment to any form of things or of life, any object, any activity; all must be renounced if need be, all must be admitted that the Divine chooses as its material for the divine life. But what accepts or rejects must be neither mind nor open or camouflaged vital will of desire nor ethical sense, but the insistence of the psychic being, the command of the Divine Guide of the Yoga, the vision of the higher Self or Spirit, the illumined guidance of the Master. The way of the spirit is not a mental way; a mental rule or mental consciousness cannot be its determinant or its leader.

Equally, a combination or a compromise between two orders of consciousness, the spiritual and the mental or the spiritual and the vital or a mere sublimation from within of Life outwardly unchanged cannot be the law or the aim of the Yoga. All life must be taken up but all life must be transformed; all must become a part, a form, an adequate expression of a spiritual being in the supramental nature. This is the height and crowning movement of a spiritual evolution in the material world, and as the change from the vital animal to mental man made life another thing altogether in basic consciousness, scope, significance, so this change from the materialised mental being to the spiritual and supramental being using but not dominated by matter must take up life and make it another thing altogether than the flawed, imperfect limited human, quite other in its basic consciousness, scope, significance. All forms of life activity that cannot bear the change must disappear, all that can bear it will survive and enter into the kingdom of the spirit. A divine Force is at work and will choose at each moment what has to be done or has not to be done, what has to be momentarily or permanently taken up, momentarily or permanently abandoned. For provided we do not substitute for that our desire or our ego, and to that end the soul must be always awake, always on guard, alive to the divine guidance, resistant to the undivine misleading from within or without us, that Force is sufficient and alone competent and she will lead us to the fulfilment along ways and by means too large, too inward, too complex for the mind to follow, much less to dictate. It is an arduous and difficult and dangerous way, but there is none other.

Two rules alone there are that will diminish the difficulty and obviate the danger. One must reject all that comes from the ego, from vital desire, from the mere mind and its presumptuous reasoning incompetence, all that ministers to these agents of the Ignorance. One must learn to hear and follow the voice of the inmost soul, the direction of the Guru, the command of the Master, the working of the Divine Mother. Whoever clings to the desires and weaknesses of the flesh, the cravings and passions of the vital in its turbulent ignorance, the dictates of his personal mind unsilenced and unillumined by a greater knowledge, cannot find the true inner law and is heaping obstacles in the way of the divine fulfilment. Whoever is able to detect and renounce those obscuring agencies and to discern and follow the true Guide within and without will discover the spiritual law and reach the goal of the Yoga.

A radical and total change of consciousness is not only the whole meaning but, in an increasing force and by progressive stages, the whole method of the integral Yoga.

---

1. *param˙ bhāvam.*
2. *mānus.īm˙ tanumāśritam.*

CHAPTER VII. STANDARDS OF CONDUCT AND SPIRITUAL FREEDOM

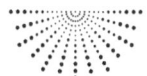

THE KNOWLEDGE on which the doer of works in Yoga has to found all his action and development has for the keystone of its structure a more and more concrete perception of unity, the living sense of an all-pervading oneness; he moves in the increasing consciousness of all existence as an indivisible whole: all work too is part of this divine indivisible whole. His personal action and its results can no longer be or seem a separate movement mainly or entirely determined by the egoistic "free" will of an individual, himself separate in the mass. Our works are part of an indivisible cosmic action; they are put or, more accurately, put themselves into their place in the whole out of which they arise and their outcome is determined by forces that overpass us. That world action in its vast totality and in every petty detail is the indivisible movement of the One who manifests himself progressively in the cosmos. Man too becomes progressively conscious of the truth of himself and the truth of things in proportion as he awakens to this One within him and outside him and to the occult, miraculous and significant process of its forces in the motion of Nature. This action, this movement, is not confined even in ourselves and those around us to the little fragmentary portion of the cosmic activities of which we in our superficial consciousness are aware; it is supported by an immense underlying environing existence subliminal to our minds or subconscious, and it is attracted by an immense transcending existence which is superconscious to our nature. Our action arises, as we ourselves have emerged, out of a universality of which we are not aware; we give it a shape by our personal temperament, personal mind and will of thought or force of impulse or desire; but the true truth of things, the true law of action exceeds these personal and human formations. Every standpoint, every man-made rule of action which ignores the indivisible totality of the cosmic movement, whatever its utility in external practice, is to the eye of spiritual Truth an imperfect view and a law of the Ignorance.

Even when we have arrived at some glimpse of this idea or succeeded in fixing it in our consciousness as a knowledge of the mind and a consequent attitude of the soul, it is difficult for us in our outward parts and active nature to square accounts between this universal standpoint and the claims of our personal opinion, our personal will, our personal emotion and desire. We are forced still to go on dealing with this indivisible movement as if it were a mass of impersonal material out of which we, the ego, the person, have to carve something according to our own will and mental fantasy by a personal struggle and effort. This is man's normal attitude towards his environment, actually false because our ego and its will are creations and puppets of the cosmic forces and it is only when we withdraw from ego into the consciousness of the divine Knowledge-Will of the Eternal who acts in them that we can be by a sort of deputation from above their master. And yet is this personal position the right attitude for man so long as he cherishes his individuality and has not yet fully developed it; for without this view-point and motive-force he cannot grow in his ego, cannot sufficiently develop and differentiate himself out of the subconscious or half-conscious universal mass-existence.

But the hold of this ego-consciousness upon our whole habit of existence is difficult to shake off when we have no longer need of the separative, the individualistic and aggressive stage of development, when we would proceed forward from this necessity of littleness in the child-soul to unity and universality, to the cosmic consciousness and beyond, to our transcendent spirit-stature. It is indispensable to recognise clearly, not only in our mode of thought but in our way of feeling, sensing, doing, that this movement, this universal action is not a helpless impersonal wave of being which lends itself to the will of any ego according to that ego's strength and insistence. It is the movement of a cosmic Being who is the Knower of his field, the steps of a Divinity who is the Master of his own progressive force of action. As the movement is one and indivisible, so he who is present in the movement is one, sole and indivisible. Not only all result is determined by him, but all initiation, action and process are dependent on the motion of his cosmic force and only belong secondarily and in their form to the creature.

But what then must be the spiritual position of the personal worker? What is his true relation in dynamic Nature to this one cosmic Being and this one total movement? He is a centre only—a centre of differentiation of the one personal consciousness, a centre of determination of the one total movement; his personality reflects in a wave of persistent individuality the one universal Person, the Transcendent, the Eternal. In the Ignorance it is always a broken and distorted reflection because the crest of the wave which is our conscious waking self throws back only an imperfect and falsified similitude of the divine Spirit. All our opinions, standards, formations, principles are only attempts to represent in this broken, reflecting and distorting mirror something of the universal and progressive total action and its many-sided movement towards some ultimate self-revelation of the Divine. Our mind represents it as best it can with a narrow approximation that becomes less and less inadequate in proportion as its thought grows in wideness and light and power; but it is always an approximation and not even a true partial figure. The Divine Will acts through the aeons to reveal progressively not only in the unity of the cosmos, not only in the collectivity of living and thinking creatures, but in the soul of each individual something of its divine Mystery and the hidden truth of the Infinite. Therefore there is in the cosmos, in the collectivity, in the individual, a rooted instinct or belief in its own perfectibility, a constant drive towards an ever increasing and more adequate and more harmonious self-development nearer to the secret truth of things. This effort is represented to the constructing mind of man by standards of knowledge, feeling, character, aesthesis and action,—rules, ideals, norms and laws that he essays to turn into universal dharmas.

If we are to be free in the spirit, if we are to be subject only to the supreme Truth, we must discard the idea that our mental or moral laws are binding on the Infinite or that there can be anything sacrosanct, absolute or eternal even in the highest of our existing standards of conduct. To form higher and higher temporary standards as long as they are needed is to serve the Divine in his world march; to erect rigidly an absolute standard is to attempt the erection of a barrier against the eternal waters in their onflow. Once the nature-bound soul realises this truth, it is delivered from the duality of good and evil. For good is all that helps the individual and the world towards their divine fullness, and evil is all that retards or breaks up that increasing perfection. But since the perfection is progressive, evolutive in Time, good and evil are also shifting quantities and change from time to time their meaning and value. This thing which is evil now and in its present shape must be abandoned was once helpful and necessary to the general and individual progress. That other thing which we now regard as evil may well become in another form and arrangement an element in some future perfection. And on the spiritual level we transcend even this distinction; for we discover the purpose and divine utility of all these things that we call good and evil. Then have we to reject the falsehood in them and all that is distorted, ignorant and obscure in that which is called good no less than in that which is called evil. For we have then to accept only the true and the divine, but to make no other distinction in the eternal processes.

To those who can act only on a rigid standard, to those who can feel only the human and not the divine values, this truth may seem to be a dangerous concession which is likely to destroy the very foundation of morality, confuse all conduct and establish only chaos. Certainly, if the choice must be between an eternal and unchanging ethics and no ethics at all, it would have that result for man in his ignorance. But even on the human level, if we have light enough and flexibility enough to recognise that a standard of conduct may be temporary and yet necessary for its time and to observe it faithfully until it can be replaced by a better, then we suffer no such loss, but lose only the fanaticism of an imperfect and intolerant virtue. In its place we gain openness and a power of continual moral progression, charity, the capacity to enter into an understanding sympathy with all this world of struggling and stumbling creatures and by that charity a better right and a greater strength to help it upon its way. In the end where the human closes and the divine commences, where the mental disappears into the supramental consciousness and the finite precipitates itself into the infinite, all evil disappears into a transcendent divine Good which becomes universal on every plane of consciousness that it touches.

This, then, stands fixed for us that all standards by which we may seek to govern our conduct are only our temporary, imperfect and evolutive attempts to represent to ourselves our stumbling mental progress in the universal self-realisation towards which Nature moves. But the divine manifestation cannot be bound by our little rules and fragile sanctities; for the consciousness behind it is too vast for these things. Once we have grasped this fact, disconcerting enough to the absolutism of our reason, we shall better be able to put in their right place in regard to each other the successive standards that govern the different stages in the growth of the individual and the collective march of mankind. At the most general of them we may cast a passing glance. For we have to see how they stand in relation to that other standardless spiritual and supramental mode of working for which Yoga seeks and to which it moves by the surrender of the individual to the divine Will and, more effectively, through his ascent by this surrender to the greater consciousness in which a certain identity with the dynamic Eternal becomes possible.

∼

There are four main standards of human conduct that make an ascending scale. The first is personal need, preference and desire; the second is the law and good of the collectivity; the third is an ideal ethic; the last is the highest divine law of the nature.

Man starts on the long career of his evolution with only the first two of these four to enlighten and lead him; for they constitute the law of his animal and vital existence and it is as the vital and physical animal man that he begins his progress. The true business of man upon earth is to express in the type of humanity a growing image of the Divine; whether knowingly or unknowingly, it is to this end that Nature is working in him under the thick veil of her inner and outer processes. But the material or animal man is ignorant of the inner aim of life; he knows only its needs and its desires and he has necessarily no other guide to what is required of him than his own perception of need and his own stirrings and pointings of desire. To satisfy his physical and vital demands and necessities before all things else and, in the next rank, whatever emotional or mental cravings or imaginations or dynamic notions rise in him must be the first natural rule of his conduct. The sole balancing or overpowering law that can modify or contradict this pressing natural claim is the demand put on him by the ideas, needs and desires of his family, community or tribe, the herd, the pack of which he is a member.

If man could live to himself,—and this he could only do if the development of the individual were the sole object of the Divine in the world,—this second law would not at all need to come into operation. But all existence proceeds by the mutual action and reaction of the whole and the parts, the need for each other of the constituents and the thing constituted, the interdependence of the group and the individuals of the group. In the language of Indian philosophy the Divine manifests himself always in the double form of the separative and the collective being, *vyaṣṭi, samaṣṭi*. Man, pressing after the growth of his separate individuality and its fullness and freedom, is unable to satisfy even his own personal needs and desires except in conjunction with other men; he is a whole in himself and yet incomplete without others. This obligation englobes his personal law of conduct in a group-law which arises from the formation of a lasting group-entity with a collective mind and life of its own to which his own embodied mind and life are subordinated as a transitory unit. And yet is there something in him immortal and free, not bound to this group-body which outlasts his own embodied existence but cannot outlast or claim to chain by its law his eternal spirit.

In itself this seemingly larger and overriding law is no more than an extension of the vital and animal principle that governs the individual elementary man; it is the law of the pack or herd. The individual identifies partially his life with the life of a certain number of other individuals with whom he is associated by birth, choice or circumstance. And since the existence of the group is necessary for his own existence and satisfaction, in time, if not from the first, its preservation, the fulfilment of its needs and the satisfaction of its collective notions, desires, habits of living, without which it would not hold together, must come to take a primary place. The satisfaction of personal idea and feeling, need and desire, propensity and habit has to be constantly subordinated, by the necessity of the situation and not from any moral or altruistic motive, to the satisfaction of the ideas and feelings, needs and desires, propensities and habits, not of this or that other individual or number of individuals, but of the society as a whole. This social need is the obscure matrix of morality and of man's ethical impulse.

It is not actually known that in any primitive times man lived to himself or with only his mate as do some of the animals. All record of him shows him to us as a social animal, not an isolated body and spirit. The law of the pack has always overridden his individual law of self-development; he seems always to have been born, to have lived, to have been formed as a unit in a mass. But logically and naturally from the psychological viewpoint the law of personal need and desire is primary, the social law comes in as a secondary and usurping power. Man has in him two distinct master impulses, the individualistic and the communal, a personal life and a social life, a personal motive of conduct and a social motive of conduct. The possibility of their opposition and the attempt to find their equation lie at the very roots of human civilisation and persist in other figures when he has passed beyond the vital animal into a highly individualised mental and spiritual progress.

The existence of a social law external to the individual is at different times a considerable advantage and a heavy disadvantage to the development of the divine in man. It is an advantage at first when man is crude and incapable of self-control and self-finding, because it erects a power other than that of his personal egoism through which that egoism may be induced or compelled to moderate its savage demands, to discipline its irrational and often violent movements and even to lose itself sometimes in a larger and less personal egoism. It is a disadvantage to the adult spirit ready to transcend the human formula because it is an external standard which seeks to impose itself on him from outside, and the condition of his perfection is that he shall grow from within and in an increasing freedom, not by the suppression but by the transcendence of his perfected individuality, not any longer by a law imposed on him that trains and disciplines his members but by the soul from within breaking through all previous forms to possess with its light and transmute his members.

～

In the conflict of the claims of society with the claims of the individual two ideal and absolute solutions confront one another. There is the demand of the group that the individual should subordinate himself more or less completely or even lose his independent existence in the community,—the smaller must be immolated or self-offered to the larger unit. He must accept the need of the society as his own need, the desire of the society as his own desire; he must live not for himself but for the tribe, clan, commune or nation of which he is a member. The ideal and absolute solution from the individual's standpoint would be a society that existed not for itself, for its all-overriding collective purpose, but for the good of the individual and his fulfilment, for the greater and more perfect life of all its members. Representing as far as possible his best self and helping him to realise it, it would respect the freedom of each of its members and maintain itself not by law and force but by the free and spontaneous consent of its constituent persons. An ideal society of either kind does not exist anywhere and would be most difficult to create, more difficult still to keep in precarious existence so long as individual man clings to his egoism as the primary motive of existence. A general but not complete domination of the society over the individual is the easier way and it is the system that Nature from the first instinctively adopts and keeps in equilibrium by rigorous law, compelling custom and a careful indoctrination of the still subservient and ill-developed intelligence of the human creature.

In primitive societies the individual life is submitted to rigid and immobile communal custom and rule; this is the ancient and would-be eternal law of the human pack that tries always to masquerade as the everlasting decree of the Imperishable, *eṣa dharmaḥ sanātanaḥ*. And the ideal is not dead in the human mind; the most recent trend of human progress is to establish an enlarged and sumptuous edition of this ancient turn of collective living towards the enslavement of the human spirit. There is here a serious danger to the integral development of a greater truth upon earth and a greater life. For the desires and free seekings of the individual, however egoistic, however false or perverted they may be in their immediate form, contain in their obscure shell the seed of a development necessary to the whole; his searchings and stumblings have behind them a force that has to be kept and transmuted into the image of the divine ideal. That force needs to be enlightened and trained but must not be suppressed or harnessed exclusively to society's heavy cartwheels. Individualism is as necessary to the final perfection as the power behind the group-spirit; the stifling of the individual may well be the stifling of the god in man. And in the present balance of humanity there is seldom any real danger of exaggerated individualism breaking up the social integer. There is continually a danger that the exaggerated pressure of the social mass by its heavy unenlightened mechanical weight may suppress or unduly discourage the free development of the individual spirit. For man in the individual can be more easily enlightened, conscious, open to clear influences; man in the mass is still obscure, half-conscious, ruled by universal forces that escape its mastery and its knowledge.

Against this danger of suppression and immobilisation Nature in the individual reacts. It may react by an isolated resistance ranging from the instinctive and brutal revolt of the criminal to the complete negation of the solitary and ascetic. It may react by the assertion of an individualistic trend in the social idea, may impose it on the mass consciousness and establish a compromise between the individual and the social demand. But a compromise is not a solution; it only salves over the difficulty and in the end increases the complexity of the problem and multiplies its issues. A new principle has to be called in other and higher than the two conflicting instincts and powerful at once to override and to reconcile them. Above the natural individual law which sets up as our one standard of conduct the satisfaction of our individual needs, preferences and desires and the natural communal law which sets up as a superior standard the satisfaction of the needs, preferences and desires of the community as a whole, there had to arise the notion of an ideal moral law which is not the satisfaction of need and desire, but controls and even coerces or annuls them in the interests of an ideal order that is not animal, not vital and physical, but mental, a creation of the mind's seeking for light and knowledge and right rule and right movement and true order. The moment this notion becomes powerful in man, he begins to escape from the engrossing vital and material into the mental life; he climbs from the first to the second degree of the threefold ascent of Nature. His needs and desires themselves are touched with a more elevated light of purpose and the mental need, the aesthetic, intellectual and emotional desire begin to predominate over the demand of the physical and vital nature.

The natural law of conduct proceeds from a conflict to an equilibrium of forces, impulsions and desires; the higher ethical law proceeds by the development of the mental and moral nature towards a fixed internal standard or else a self-formed ideal of absolute qualities,—justice, righteousness, love, right reason, right power, beauty, light. It is therefore essentially an individual standard; it is not a creation of the mass mind. The thinker is the individual; it is he who calls out and throws into forms that which would otherwise remain subconscious in the amorphous human whole. The moral striver is also the individual; self-discipline, not under the yoke of an outer law, but in obedience to an internal light, is essentially an individual effort. But by positing his personal standard as the translation of an absolute moral ideal the thinker imposes it, not on himself alone, but on all the individuals whom his thought can reach and penetrate. And as the mass of individuals come more and more to accept it in idea if only in an imperfect practice or no practice, society also is compelled to obey the new orientation. It absorbs the ideative influence and tries, not with any striking success, to mould its institutions into new forms touched by these higher ideals. But always its instinct is to translate them into binding law, into pattern forms, into mechanic custom, into an external social compulsion upon its living units.

For, long after the individual has become partially free, a moral organism capable of conscious growth, aware of an inward life, eager for spiritual progress, society continues to be external in its methods, a material and economic organism, mechanical, more intent upon status and self-preservation than on growth and self-perfection. The greatest present triumph of the thinking and progressive individual over the instinctive and static society has been the power he has acquired by his thought-will to compel it to think also, to open itself to the idea of social justice and righteousness, communal sympathy and mutual compassion, to feel after the rule of reason rather than blind custom as the test of its institutions and to look on the mental and moral assent of its individuals as at least one essential element in the validity of its laws. Ideally at least, to consider light rather than force as its sanction, moral development and not vengeance or restraint as the object even of its penal action, is becoming just possible to the communal mind. The greatest future triumph of the thinker will come when he can persuade the individual integer and the collective whole to rest their life-relation and its union and stability upon a free and harmonious consent and self-adaptation, and shape and govern the external by the internal truth rather than to constrain the inner spirit by the tyranny of the external form and structure.

But even this success that he has gained is rather a thing in potentiality than in actual accomplishment. There is always a disharmony and a discord between the moral law in the individual and the law of his needs and desires, between the moral law proposed to society and the physical and vital needs, desires, customs, prejudices, interests and passions of the caste, the clan, the religious community, the society, the nation. The moralist erects in vain his absolute ethical standard and calls upon all to be faithful to it without regard to consequences. To him the needs and desires of the individual are invalid if they are in conflict with the moral law, and the social law has no claims upon him if it is opposed to his sense of right and denied by his conscience. This is his absolute solution for the individual that he shall cherish no desires and claims that are not consistent with love, truth and justice. He demands from the community or nation that it shall hold all things cheap, even its safety and its most pressing interests, in comparison with truth, justice, humanity and the highest good of the peoples.

No individual rises to these heights except in intense moments, no society yet created satisfies this ideal. And in the present state of morality and of human development none perhaps can or ought to satisfy it. Nature will not allow it, Nature knows that it should not be. The first reason is that our moral ideals are themselves for the most part ill-evolved, ignorant and arbitrary, mental construction rather than transcriptions of the eternal truths of the spirit. Authoritative and dogmatic, they assert certain absolute standards in theory, but in practice every existing system of ethics proves either in application unworkable or is in fact a constant coming short of the absolute standard to which the ideal pretends. If our ethical system is a compromise or a makeshift, it gives at once a principle of justification to the further sterilising compromises which society and the individual hasten to make with it. And if it insists on absolute love, justice, right with an uncompromising insistence, it soars above the head of human possibility and is professed with lip homage but ignored in practice. Even it is found that it ignores other elements in humanity which equally insist on survival but refuse to come within the moral formula. For just as the individual law of desire contains within it invaluable elements of the infinite whole which have to be protected against the tyranny of the absorbing social idea, the innate impulses too both of individual and of collective man contain in them invaluable elements which escape the limits of any ethical formula yet discovered and are yet necessary to the fullness and harmony of an eventual divine perfection.

Moreover, absolute love, absolute justice, absolute right reason in their present application by a bewildered and imperfect humanity come easily to be conflicting principles. Justice often demands what love abhors. Right reason dispassionately considering the facts of nature and human relations in search of a satisfying norm or rule is unable to admit without modification either any reign of absolute justice or any reign of absolute love. And in fact man's absolute justice easily turns out to be in practice a sovereign injustice; for his mind, one-sided and rigid in its constructions, puts forward a one-sided partial and rigorous scheme or figure and claims for it totality and absoluteness and an application that ignores the subtler truth of things and the plasticity of life. All our standards turned into action either waver on a flux of compromises or err by this partiality and unelastic structure. Humanity sways from one orientation to another; the race moves upon a zigzag path led by conflicting claims and, on the whole, works out instinctively what Nature intends, but with much waste and suffering, rather than either what it desires or what it holds to be right or what the highest light from above demands from the embodied spirit.

∽

The fact is that when we have reached the cult of absolute ethical qualities and erected the categorical imperative of an ideal law, we have not come to the end of our search or touched the truth that delivers. There is, no doubt, something here that helps us to rise beyond limitation by the physical and vital man in us, an insistence that overpasses the individual and collective needs and desires of a humanity still bound to the living mud of Matter in which it took its roots, an aspiration that helps to develop the mental and moral being in us: this new sublimating element has been therefore an acquisition of great importance; its workings have marked a considerable step forward in the difficult evolution of terrestrial Nature. And behind the inadequacy of these ethical conceptions something too is concealed that does attach to a supreme Truth; there is here the glimmer of a light and power that are part of a yet unreached divine Nature. But the mental idea of these things is not that light and the moral formulation of them is not that power. These are only representative constructions of the mind that cannot embody the divine spirit which they vainly endeavour to imprison in their categorical formulas. Beyond the mental and moral being in us is a greater divine being that is spiritual and supramental; for it is only through a large spiritual plane where the mind's formulas dissolve in a white flame of direct inner experience that we can reach beyond mind and pass from its constructions to the vastness and freedom of the supramental realities. There alone can we touch the harmony of the divine powers that are poorly mispresented to our mind or framed into a false figure by the conflicting or wavering elements of the moral law. There alone the unification of the transformed vital and physical and the illumined mental man becomes possible in that supramental Spirit which is at once the secret source and goal of our mind and life and body. There alone is there any possibility of an absolute justice, love and right—far other than that which we imagine—at one with each other in the light of a supreme divine knowledge. There alone can there be a reconciliation of the conflict between our members.

In other words there is, above society's external law and man's moral law and beyond them, though feebly and ignorantly aimed at by something within them, a larger truth of a vast unbound consciousness, a law divine towards which both these blind and gross formulations are progressive faltering steps that try to escape from the natural law of the animal to a more exalted light or universal rule. That divine standard, since the godhead in us is our spirit moving towards its own concealed perfection, must be a supreme spiritual law and truth of our nature. Again, as we are embodied beings in the world with a common existence and nature and yet individual souls capable of direct touch with the Transcendent, this supreme truth of ourselves must have a double character. It must be a law and truth that discovers the perfect movement, harmony, rhythm of a great spiritualised collective life and determines perfectly our relations with each being and all beings in Nature's varied oneness. It must be at the same time a law and truth that discovers to us at each moment the rhythm and exact steps of the direct expression of the Divine in the soul, mind, life, body of the individual creature.[1] And we find in experience that this supreme light and force of action in its highest expression is at once an imperative law and an absolute freedom. It is an imperative law because it governs by immutable Truth our every inner and outer movement. And yet at each moment and in each movement the absolute freedom of the Supreme handles the perfect plasticity of our conscious and liberated nature.

The ethical idealist tries to discover this supreme law in his own moral data, in the inferior powers and factors that belong to the mental and ethical formula. And to sustain and organise them he selects a fundamental principle of conduct essentially unsound and constructed by the intellect—utility, hedonism, reason, intuitive conscience or any other generalised standard. All such efforts are foredoomed to failure. Our inner nature is the progressive expression of the eternal Spirit and too complex a power to be tied down by a single dominant mental or moral principle. Only the supramental consciousness can reveal to its differing and conflicting forces their spiritual truth and harmonise their divergences.

The later religions endeavour to fix the type of a supreme truth of conduct, erect a system and declare God's law through the mouth of Avatar or prophet. These systems, more powerful and dynamic than the dry ethical idea, are yet for the most part no more than idealistic glorifications of the moral principle sanctified by religious emotion and the label of a superhuman origin. Some, like the extreme Christian ethic, are rejected by Nature because they insist unworkably on an impracticable absolute rule. Others prove in the end to be evolutionary compromises and become obsolete in the march of Time. The true divine law, unlike these mental counterfeits, cannot be a system of rigid ethical determinations that press into their cast-iron moulds all our life-movements. The Law divine is truth of life and truth of the spirit and must take up with a free living plasticity and inspire with the direct touch of its eternal light each step of our action and all the complexity of our life issues. It must act not as a rule and formula but as an enveloping and penetrating conscious presence that determines all our thoughts, activities, feelings, impulses of will by its infallible power and knowledge.

The older religions erected their rule of the wise, their dicta of Manu or Confucius, a complex Shastra in which they attempted to combine the social rule and moral law with the declaration of certain eternal principles of our highest nature in some kind of uniting amalgam. All three were treated on the same ground as equally the expression of everlasting verities, *sanātana dharma*. But two of these elements are evolutionary and valid for a time, mental constructions, human readings of the will of the Eternal; the third, attached and subdued to certain social and moral formulas, had to share the fortunes of its forms. Either the Shastra grows obsolete and has to be progressively changed or finally cast away or else it stands as a rigid barrier to the self-development of the individual and the race. The Shastra erects a collective and external standard; it ignores the inner nature of the individual, the indeterminable elements of a secret spiritual force within him. But the nature of the individual will not be ignored; its demand is inexorable. The unrestrained indulgence of his outer impulses leads to anarchy and dissolution, but the suppression and coercion of his soul's freedom by a fixed and mechanical rule spells stagnation or an inner death. Not this coercion or determination from outside, but the free discovery of his highest spirit and the truth of an eternal movement is the supreme thing that he has to discover.

The higher ethical law is discovered by the individual in his mind and will and psychic sense and then extended to the race. The supreme law also must be discovered by the individual in his spirit. Then only, through a spiritual influence and not by the mental idea, can it be extended to others. A moral law can be imposed as a rule or an ideal on numbers of men who have not attained that level of consciousness or that fineness of mind and will and psychic sense in which it can become a reality to them and a living force. As an ideal it can be revered without any need of practice. As a rule it can be observed in its outsides even if the inner sense is missed altogether. The supramental and spiritual life cannot be mechanised in this way, it cannot be turned into a mental ideal or an external rule. It has its own great lines, but these must be made real, must be the workings of an active Power felt in the individual's consciousness and the transcriptions of an eternal Truth powerful to transform mind, life and body. And because it is thus real, effective, imperative, the generalisation of the supramental consciousness and the spiritual life is the sole force that can lead to individual and collective perfection in earth's highest creatures. Only by our coming into constant touch with the divine Consciousness and its absolute Truth can some form of the conscious Divine, the dynamic Absolute, take up our earth-existence and transform its strife, stumbling, sufferings and falsities into an image of the supreme Light, Power and Ananda.

The culmination of the soul's constant touch with the Supreme is that self-giving which we call surrender to the divine Will and immergence of the separated ego in the One who is all. A vast universality of soul and an intense unity with all is the base and fixed condition of the supramental consciousness and spiritual life. In that universality and unity alone can we find the supreme law of the divine manifestation in the life of the embodied spirit; in that alone can we discover the supreme motion and right play of our individual nature. In that alone can all these lower discords resolve themselves into a victorious harmony of the true relations between manifested beings who are portions of the one Godhead and children of one universal Mother.

~

All conduct and action are part of the movement of a Power, a Force infinite and divine in its origin and secret sense and will even though the forms of it we see seem inconscient or ignorant, material, vital, mental, finite, which is working to bring out progressively something of the Divine and Infinite in the obscurity of the individual and collective nature. This power is leading towards the Light, but still through the Ignorance. It leads man first through his needs and desires; it guides him next through enlarged needs and desires modified and enlightened by a mental and moral ideal. It is preparing to lead him to a spiritual realisation that overrides these things and yet fulfils and reconciles them in all that is divinely true in their spirit and purpose. It transforms the needs and desires into a divine Will and Ananda. It transforms the mental and moral aspiration into the powers of Truth and Perfection that are beyond them. It substitutes for the divided straining of the individual nature, for the passion and strife of the separate ego, the calm, profound, harmonious and happy law of the universalised person within us, the central being, the spirit that is a portion of the supreme Spirit. This true Person in us, because it is universal, does not seek its separate gratification but only asks in its outward expression in Nature its growth to its real stature, the expression of its inner divine self, that transcendent spiritual power and presence within it which is one with all and in sympathy with each thing and creature and with all the collective personalities and powers of the divine existence, and yet it transcends them and is not bound by the egoism of any creature or collectivity or limited by the ignorant controls of their lower nature. This is the high realisation in front of all our seeking and striving, and it gives the sure promise of a perfect reconciliation and transmutation of all the elements of our nature. A pure, total and flawless action is possible only when that is effected and we have reached the height of this secret Godhead within us.

The perfect supramental action will not follow any single principle or limited rule. It is not likely to satisfy the standard either of the individual egoist or of any organised group-mind. It will conform to the demand neither of the positive practical man of the world nor of the formal moralist nor of the patriot nor of the sentimental philanthropist nor of the idealising philosopher. It will proceed by a spontaneous outflowing from the summits in the totality of an illumined and uplifted being, will and knowledge and not by the selected, calculated and standardised action which is all that the intellectual reason or ethical will can achieve. Its sole aim will be the expression of the divine in us and the keeping together of the world and its progress towards the Manifestation that is to be. This even will not be so much an aim and purpose as a spontaneous law of the being and an intuitive determination of the action by the Light of the divine Truth and its automatic influence. It will proceed like the action of Nature from a total will and knowledge behind her, but a will and knowledge enlightened in a conscious supreme Nature and no longer obscure in this ignorant Prakriti. It will be an action not bound by the dualities but full and large in the spirit's impartial joy of existence. The happy and inspired movement of a divine Power and Wisdom guiding and impelling us will replace the perplexities and stumblings of the suffering and ignorant ego.

If by some miracle of divine intervention all mankind at once could be raised to this level, we should have something on earth like the Golden Age of the traditions, Satya Yuga, the Age of Truth or true existence. For the sign of the Satya Yuga is that the Law is spontaneous and conscious in each creature and does its own works in a perfect harmony and freedom. Unity and universality, not separative division, would be the foundation of the consciousness of the race; love would be absolute; equality would be consistent with hierarchy and perfect in difference; absolute justice would be secured by the spontaneous action of the being in harmony with the truth of things and the truth of himself and others and therefore sure of true and right result; right reason, no longer mental but supramental, would be satisfied not by the observation of artificial standards but by the free automatic perception of right relations and their inevitable execution in the act. The quarrel between the individual and society or disastrous struggle between one community and another could not exist: the cosmic consciousness imbedded in embodied beings would assure a harmonious diversity in oneness.

In the actual state of humanity, it is the individual who must climb to this height as a pioneer and precursor. His isolation will necessarily give a determination and a form to his outward activities that must be quite other than those of a consciously divine collective action. The inner state, the root of his acts, will be the same; but the acts themselves may well be very different from what they would be on an earth liberated from ignorance. Nevertheless his consciousness and the divine mechanism of his conduct, if such a word can be used of so free a thing, would be such as has been described, free from that subjection to vital impurity and desire and wrong impulse which we call sin, unbound by that rule of prescribed moral formulas which we call virtue, spontaneously sure and pure and perfect in a greater consciousness than the mind's, governed in all its steps by the light and truth of the Spirit. But if a collectivity or group could be formed of those who had reached the supramental perfection, there indeed some divine creation could take shape; a new earth could descend that would be a new heaven, a world of supramental light could be created here amidst the receding darkness of this terrestrial ignorance.

---

1. Therefore the Gita defines "dharma", an expression which means more than either religion or morality, as action controlled by our essential manner of self-being.

CHAPTER VIII. THE SUPREME WILL

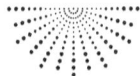

IN THE light of this progressive manifestation of the Spirit, first apparently bound in the Ignorance, then free in the power and wisdom of the Infinite, we can better understand the great and crowning injunction of the Gita to the Karmayogin, "Abandoning all dharmas, all principles and laws and rules of conduct, take refuge in me alone." All standards and rules are temporary constructions founded upon the needs of the ego in its transition from Matter to Spirit. These makeshifts have a relative imperativeness so long as we rest satisfied in the stages of transition, content with the physical and vital life, attached to the mental movement, or even fixed in the ranges of the mental plane that are touched by the spiritual lustres. But beyond is the unwalled wideness of a supramental infinite consciousness and there all temporary structures cease. It is not possible to enter utterly into the spiritual truth of the Eternal and Infinite if we have not the faith and courage to trust ourselves into the hands of the Lord of all things and the Friend of all creatures and leave utterly behind us our mental limits and measures. At one moment we must plunge without hesitation, reserve, fear or scruple into the ocean of the free, the infinite, the Absolute. After the Law, Liberty; after the personal, after the general, after the universal standards there is something greater, the impersonal plasticity, the divine freedom, the transcendent force and the supernal impulse. After the strait path of the ascent the wide plateaus on the summit.

There are three stages of the ascent,—at the bottom the bodily life enslaved to the pressure of necessity and desire, in the middle the mental, higher emotional and psychic rule that feels after greater interests, aspirations, experiences, at the summits first a deeper psychic and spiritual state and then a supramental eternal consciousness in which all our aspirations and seekings discover their own intimate significance. In the bodily life first desire and need and then the practical good of the individual and the society are the governing consideration, the dominant force. In the mental life ideas and ideals rule, ideas that are half-lights wearing the garb of Truth, ideals formed by the mind as a result of a growing but still imperfect intuition and experience. Whenever the mental life prevails and the bodily diminishes its brute insistence, man the mental being feels pushed by the urge of mental Nature to mould in the sense of the idea or the ideal the life of the individual, and in the end even the vaguer more complex life of the society is forced to undergo this subtle process. In the spiritual life, or when a higher power than Mind has manifested and taken possession of the nature, these limited motive-forces recede, dwindle, tend to disappear. The spiritual or supramental Self, the Divine Being, the supreme and immanent Reality, must be alone the Lord within us and shape freely our final development according to the highest, widest, most integral expression possible of the law of our nature. In the end that nature acts in the perfect Truth and its spontaneous freedom; for it obeys only the luminous power of the Eternal. The individual has nothing further to gain, no desire to fulfil; he has become a portion of the impersonality or the universal personality of the Eternal. No other object than the manifestation and play of the Divine Spirit in life and the maintenance and conduct of the world in its march towards the divine goal can move him to action. Mental ideas, opinions, constructions are his no more; for his mind has fallen into silence, it is only a channel for the Light and Truth of the divine knowledge. Ideals are too narrow for the vastness of his spirit; it is the ocean of the Infinite that flows through him and moves him for ever.

Whoever sincerely enters the path of works, must leave behind him the stage in which need and desire are the first law of our acts. For whatever desires still trouble his being, he must, if he accepts the high aim of Yoga, put them away from him into the hands of the Lord within us. The supreme Power will deal with them for the good of the sadhaka and for the good of all. In effect, we find that once this surrender is done,—always provided the rejection is sincere,—egoistic indulgence of desire may for some time recur under the continued impulse of past nature but only in order to exhaust its acquired momentum and to teach the embodied being in his most unteachable part, his nervous, vital, emotional nature, by the reactions of desire, by its grief and unrest bitterly contrasted with calm periods of the higher peace or marvellous movements of divine Ananda, that egoistic desire is not a law for the soul that seeks liberation or aspires to its own original god-nature. Afterwards the element of desire in those impulsions will be thrown away or persistently eliminated by a constant denying and transforming pressure. Only the pure force of action in them (*pravṛtti*) justified by an equal delight in all work and result that is inspired or imposed from above will be preserved in the happy harmony of a final perfection. To act, to enjoy is the normal law and right of the nervous being; but to choose by personal desire its action and enjoyment is only its ignorant will, not its right. Alone the supreme and universal Will must choose; action must change into a dynamic movement of that Will; enjoyment must be replaced by the play of a pure spiritual Ananda. All personal will is either a temporary delegation from on high or a usurpation by the ignorant Asura.

The social law, that second term of our progress, is a means to which the ego is subjected in order that it may learn discipline by subordination to a wider collective ego. This law may be quite empty of any moral content and may express only the needs or the practical good of the society as each society conceives it. Or it may express those needs and that good, but modified and coloured and supplemented by a higher moral or ideal law. It is binding on the developing but not yet perfectly developed individual in the shape of social duty, family obligation, communal or national demand, so long as it is not in conflict with his growing sense of the higher Right. But the sadhaka of the Karmayoga will abandon this also to the Lord of works. After he has made this surrender, his social impulses and judgments will, like his desires, only be used for their exhaustion or, it may be, so far as they are still necessary for a time to enable him to identify his lower mental nature with mankind in general or with any grouping of mankind in its works and hopes and aspirations. But after that brief time is over, they will be withdrawn and a divine government will alone abide. He will be identified with the Divine and with others only through the divine consciousness and not through the mental nature.

For, even after he is free, the sadhaka will be in the world and to be in the world is to remain in works. But to remain in works without desire is to act for the good of the world in general or for the kind or the race or for some new creation to be evolved on the earth or some work imposed by the Divine Will within him. And this must be done either in the framework provided by the environment or the grouping in which he is born or placed or else in one which is chosen or created for him by a divine direction. Therefore in our perfection there must be nothing left in the mental being which conflicts with or prevents our sympathy and free self-identification with the kind, the group or whatever collective expression of the Divine he is meant to lead, help or serve. But in the end it must become a free self-identification through identity with the Divine and not a mental bond or moral tie of union or a vital association dominated by any kind of personal, social, national, communal or credal egoism. If any social law is obeyed, it will not be from physical necessity or from the sense of personal or general interest or for expediency or because of the pressure of the environment or from any sense of duty, but solely for the sake of the Lord of works and because it is felt or known to be the Divine Will that the social law or rule or relation as it stands can still be kept as a figure of the inner life and the minds of men must not be disturbed by its infringement. If, on the other hand, the social law, rule or relation is disregarded, that too will not be for the indulgence of desire, personal will or personal opinion, but because a greater rule is felt that expresses the law of the Spirit or because it is known that there must be in the march of the divine All-Will a movement towards the changing, exceeding or abolition of existing laws and forms for the sake of a freer larger life necessary to the world's progress.

There is still left the moral law or the ideal and these, even to many who think themselves free, appear for ever sacred and intangible. But the sadhaka, his gaze turned always to the heights, will abandon them to Him whom all ideals seek imperfectly and fragmentarily to express; all moral qualities are only a poor and rigid travesty of his spontaneous and illimitable perfection. The bondage to sin and evil passes away with the passing of nervous desire; for it belongs to the quality of vital passion, impulsion or drive of propensity in us (*rajoguṇa*) and is extinguished with the transformation of that mode of Nature. But neither must the aspirant remain subject to the gilded or golden chain of a conventional or a habitual or a mentally ordered or even a high or clear sattwic virtue. That will be replaced by something profounder and more essential than the minor inadequate thing that men call virtue. The original sense of the word was manhood and this is a much larger and deeper thing than the moral mind and its structures. The culmination of Karmayoga is a yet higher and deeper state that may perhaps be called "soul-hood",—for the soul is greater than the man; a free soul-hood spontaneously welling out in works of a supreme Truth and Love will replace human virtue. But this supreme Truth cannot be forced to inhabit the petty edifices of the practical reason or even confined in the more dignified constructions of the larger ideative reason that imposes its representations as if they were pure truth on the limited human intelligence. This supreme Love will not necessarily be consistent, much less will it be synonymous, with the partial and feeble, ignorant and emotion-ridden movements of human attraction, sympathy and pity. The petty law cannot bind the vaster movement; the mind's partial attainment cannot dictate its terms to the soul's supreme fulfilment.

At first, the higher Love and Truth will fulfil its movement in the sadhaka according to the essential law or way of his own nature. For that is the special aspect of the divine Nature, the particular power of the supreme Shakti, out of which his soul has emerged into the Play, not limited indeed by the forms of this law or way, for the soul is infinite. But still its stuff of nature bears that stamp, evolves fluently along those lines or turns around the spiral curves of that dominating influence. He will manifest the divine Truth-movement according to the temperament of the sage or the lion-like fighter or the lover and enjoyer or the worker and servant or in any combination of essential attributes (gunas) that may constitute the form given to his being by its own inner urge. It is this self-nature playing freely in his acts which men will see in him and not a conduct cut, chalked out, artificially regulated, by any lesser rule or by any law from outside.

But there is a yet higher attainment, there is an infinity (*ānantya*) in which even this last limitation is exceeded, because the nature is utterly fulfilled and its boundaries vanish. There the soul lives without any boundaries; for it uses all forms and moulds according to the divine Will in it, but it is not restrained, it is not tied down, it is not imprisoned in any power or form that it uses. This is the summit of the path of works and this the utter liberty of the soul in its actions. In reality, it has there no actions; for all its activities are a rhythm of the Supreme and sovereignly proceed from That alone like a spontaneous music out of the Infinite.

The total surrender, then, of all our actions to a supreme and universal Will, an unconditioned and standardless surrender of all works to the government of something eternal within us which will replace the ordinary working of the ego-nature, is the way and end of Karmayoga. But what is this divine supreme Will and how can it be recognised by our deluded instruments and our blind prisoned intelligence?

Ordinarily, we conceive of ourselves as a separate "I" in the universe that governs a separate body and mental and moral nature, chooses in full liberty its own self-determined actions and is independent and therefore sole master of its works and responsible. It is not easy for the ordinary mind, the mind that has not thought nor looked deeply into its own constitution and constituents, it is difficult even for minds that have thought but have no spiritual vision and experience, to imagine how there can be anything else in us truer, deeper and more powerful than this apparent "I" and its empire. But the very first step towards self-knowledge as towards the true knowledge of phenomena is to get behind the apparent truth of things and find the real but masked, essential and dynamic truth which their appearances cover.

This ego or "I" is not a lasting truth, much less our essential part; it is only a formation of Nature, a mental form of thought-centralisation in the perceiving and discriminating mind, a vital form of the centralisation of feeling and sensation in our parts of life, a form of physical conscious reception centralising substance and function of substance in our bodies. All that we internally are is not ego, but consciousness, soul or spirit. All that we externally and superficially are and do is not ego but Nature. An executive cosmic force shapes us and dictates through our temperament and environment and mentality so shaped, through our individualised formulation of the cosmic energies, our actions and their results. Truly, we do not think, will or act but thought occurs in us, will occurs in us, impulse and act occur in us; our ego-sense gathers around itself, refers to itself all this flow of natural activities. It is cosmic Force, it is Nature that forms the thought, imposes the will, imparts the impulse. Our body, mind and ego are a wave of that sea of force in action and do not govern it, but by it are governed and directed. The sadhaka in his progress towards truth and self-knowledge must come to a point where the soul opens its eyes of vision and recognises this truth of ego and this truth of works. He gives up the idea of a mental, vital, physical "I" that acts or governs action; he recognises that Prakriti, Force of cosmic nature following her fixed modes, is the one and only worker in him and in all things and creatures.

But what has fixed the modes of Nature? Or who has originated and governs the movements of Force? There is a Consciousness—or a Conscient—behind that is the lord, witness, knower, enjoyer, upholder and source of sanction for her works; this consciousness is Soul or Purusha. Prakriti shapes the action in us; Purusha in her or behind her witnesses, assents, bears and upholds it. Prakriti forms the thought in our minds; Purusha in her or behind her knows the thought and the truth in it. Prakriti determines the result of the action; Purusha in her or behind her enjoys or suffers the consequence. Prakriti forms mind and body, labours over them, develops them; Purusha upholds the formation and evolution and sanctions each step of her works. Prakriti applies the Will-force which works in things and men; Purusha sets that Will-force to work by his vision of that which should be done. This Purusha is not the surface ego, but a silent Self, a source of Power, an originator and receiver of Knowledge behind the ego. Our mental "I" is only a false reflection of this Self, this Power, this Knowledge. This Purusha or supporting Consciousness is therefore the cause, recipient and support of all Nature's works, but he is not himself the doer. Prakriti, NatureForce, in front and Shakti, Conscious-Force, Soul-Force behind her,—for these two are the inner and outer faces of the universal Mother,—account for all that is done in the universe. The universal Mother, Prakriti-Shakti, is the one and only worker.

Purusha-Prakriti, Consciousness-Force, Soul supporting Nature,—for the two even in their separation are one and inseparable,—are at once a universal and a transcendent Power. But there is something in the individual too which is not the mental ego, something that is one in essence with this greater reality: it is a pure reflection or portion of the one Purusha; it is the Soul Person or the embodied being, the individual self, Jivatman; it is the Self that seems to limit its power and knowledge so as to support an individual play of transcendent and universal Nature. In deepest reality the infinitely One is also infinitely multiple; we are not only a reflection or portion of That but we are That; our spiritual individuality —unlike our ego—does not preclude our universality and transcendence. But at present the soul or self in us intent on individualisation in Nature allows itself to be confused with the idea of the ego; it has to get rid of this ignorance, it has to know itself as a reflection or portion or being of the supreme and universal Self and solely a centre of its consciousness in the world-action. But this Jiva Purusha too is not the doer of works any more than the ego or the supporting consciousness of the Witness and Knower. Again and always it is the transcendent and universal Shakti who is the sole doer. But behind her is the one Supreme who manifests through her as the dual power, Purusha-Prakriti, Ishwara-Shakti.[1] The Supreme becomes dynamic as the Shakti and is by her the sole originator and Master of works in the universe.

If this is the truth of works, the first thing the sadhaka has to do is to recoil from the egoistic forms of activity and get rid of the sense of an "I" that acts. He has to see and feel that everything happens in him by the plastic conscious or subconscious or sometimes superconscious automatism of his mental and bodily instruments moved by the forces of spiritual, mental, vital and physical Nature. There is a personality on his surface that chooses and wills, submits and struggles, tries to make good in Nature or prevail over Nature, but this personality is itself a construction of Nature and so dominated, driven, determined by her that it cannot be free. It is a formation or expression of the Self in her,—it is a self of Nature rather than a self of Self, his natural and processive, not his spiritual and permanent being, a temporary constructed personality, not the true immortal Person. It is that Person that he must become. He must succeed in being inwardly quiescent, detach himself as the observer from the outer active personality and learn the play of the cosmic forces in him by standing back from all blinding absorption in its turns and movements. Thus calm, detached, a student of himself and a witness of his nature, he realises that he is the individual soul who observes the works of Nature, accepts tranquilly her results and sanctions or withholds his sanction from the impulse to her acts. At present this soul or Purusha is little more than an acquiescent spectator, influencing perhaps the action and development of the being by the pressure of its veiled consciousness, but for the most part delegating its powers or a fragment of them to the outer personality,—in fact to Nature, for this outer self is not lord but subject to her, *anīśa*; but, once unveiled, it can make its sanction or refusal effective, become the master of the action, dictate sovereignly a change of Nature. Even if for a long time, as the result of fixed association and past storage of energy, the habitual movement takes place independent of the Purusha's assent and even if the sanctioned movement is persistently refused by Nature for want of past habit, still he will discover that in the end his assent or refusal prevails,—slowly with much resistance or quickly with a rapid accommodation of her means and tendencies she modifies herself and her workings in the direction indicated by his inner sight or volition. Thus he learns in place of mental control or egoistic will an inner spiritual control which makes him master of the Nature-forces that work in him and not their unconscious instrument or mechanic slave. Above and around him is the Shakti, the universal Mother and from her he can get all his inmost soul needs and wills if only he has a true knowledge of her ways and a true surrender to the divine Will in her. Finally, he becomes aware of that highest dynamic Self within him and within Nature which is the source of all his seeing and knowing, the source of the sanction, the source of the acceptance, the source of the rejection. This is the Lord, the Supreme, the One-in-all, Ishwara-Shakti, of whom his soul is a portion, a being of that Being and a power of that Power. The rest of our progress depends on our knowledge of the ways in which the Lord of works manifests his Will in the world and in us and executes them through the transcendent and universal Shakti.

The Lord sees in his omniscience the thing that has to be done. This seeing is his Will, it is a form of creative Power, and that which he sees the all-conscious Mother, one with him, takes into her dynamic self and embodies, and executive Nature-Force carries it out as the mechanism of their omnipotent omniscience. But this vision of what is to be and therefore of what is to be done arises out of the very being, pours directly out of the consciousness and delight of existence of the Lord, spontaneously, like light from the Sun. It is not our mortal attempt to see, our difficult arrival at truth of action and motive or just demand of Nature. When the individual soul is entirely at one in its being and knowledge with the Lord and directly in touch with the original Shakti, the transcendent Mother, the supreme Will can then arise in us too in the high divine manner as a thing that must be and is achieved by the spontaneous action of Nature. There is then no desire, no responsibility, no reaction; all takes place in the peace, calm, light, power of the supporting and enveloping and inhabiting Divine.

But even before that highest approach to identity is achieved, something of the supreme Will can manifest in us as an imperative impulsion, a God-driven action; we then act by a spontaneous self-determining Force but a fuller knowledge of meaning and aim arises only afterwards. Or the impulse to action may come as an inspiration or intuition, but rather in the heart and body than in the mind; here an effective sight enters in but the complete and exact knowledge is still deferred and comes, if at all, later. But the divine Will may descend too as a luminous single command or a total perception or a continuous current of perception of what is to be done into the will or into the thought or as a direction from above spontaneously fulfilled by the lower members. When the Yoga is imperfect, only some actions can be done in this way, or else a general action may so proceed but only during periods of exaltation and illumination. When the Yoga is perfect, all action becomes of this character. We may indeed distinguish three stages of a growing progress by which, first, the personal will is occasionally or frequently enlightened or moved by a supreme Will or conscious Force beyond it, then constantly replaced and, last, identified and merged in that divine Power-action. The first is the stage when we are still governed by the intellect, heart and senses; these have to seek or wait for the divine inspiration and guidance and do not always find or receive it. The second is the stage when human intelligence is more and more replaced by a high illumined or intuitive spiritualised mind, the external human heart by the inner psychic heart, the senses by a purified and selfless vital force. The third is the stage when we rise even above spiritualised mind to the supramental levels.

In all three stages the fundamental character of the liberated action is the same, a spontaneous working of Prakriti no longer through or for the ego but at the will and for the enjoyment of the supreme Purusha. At a higher level this becomes the Truth of the absolute and universal Supreme expressed through the individual soul and worked out consciously through the nature,—no longer through a half-perception and a diminished or distorted effectuation by the stumbling, ignorant and all-deforming energy of lower nature in us but by the all-wise transcendent and universal Mother.

The Lord has veiled himself and his absolute wisdom and eternal consciousness in ignorant Nature-Force and suffers her to drive the individual being, with its complicity, as the ego; this lower action of Nature continues to prevail, often even in spite of man's half-lit imperfect efforts at a nobler motive and a purer self-knowledge. Our human effort at perfection fails, or progresses very incompletely, owing to the force of Nature's past actions in us, her past formations, her long-rooted associations; it turns towards a true and high-climbing success only when a greater Knowledge and Power than our own breaks through the lid of our ignorance and guides or takes up our personal will. For our human will is a misled and wandering ray that has parted from the supreme Puissance. The period of slow emergence out of this lower working into a higher light and purer force is the valley of the shadow of death for the striver after perfection; it is a dreadful passage full of trials, sufferings, sorrows, obscurations, stumblings, errors, pitfalls. To abridge and alleviate this ordeal or to penetrate it with the divine delight faith is necessary, an increasing surrender of the mind to the knowledge that imposes itself from within and, above all, a true aspiration and a right and unfaltering and sincere practice. "Practise unfalteringly," says the Gita, "with a heart free from despondency," the Yoga; for even though in the earlier stage of the path we drink deep of the bitter poison of internal discord and suffering, the last taste of this cup is the sweetness of the nectar of immortality and the honey-wine of an eternal Ananda.

---

1. Ishwara-Shakti is not quite the same as Purusha-Prakriti; for Purusha and Prakriti are separate powers, but Ishwara and Shakti contain each other. Ishwara is Purusha who contains Prakriti and rules by the power of the Shakti within him. Shakti is Prakriti ensouled by Purusha and acts by the will of the Ishwara which is her own will and whose presence in her movement she carries always with her. The Purusha-Prakriti realisation is of the first utility to the seeker on the Way of Works; for it is the separation of the conscient being and the Energy and the subjection of the being to the mechanism of the Energy that are the efficient cause of our ignorance and imperfection; by this realisation the being can liberate himself from the mechanical action of the nature and become free and arrive at a first spiritual control over the nature. Ishwara-Shakti stands behind the relation of Purusha-Prakriti and its ignorant action and turns it to an evolutionary purpose. The Ishwara-Shakti realisation can bring participation in a higher dynamism and a divine working and a total unity and harmony of the being in a spiritual nature.

CHAPTER IX. EQUALITY AND THE ANNIHILATION OF EGO

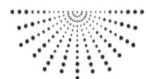

AN ENTIRE self-consecration, a complete equality, an unsparing effacement of the ego, a transforming deliverance of the nature from its ignorant modes of action are the steps by which the surrender of all the being and nature to the Divine Will can be prepared and achieved,—a self-giving true, total and without reserve. The first necessity is an entire spirit of self-consecration in our works; it must become first the constant will, then the ingrained need in all the being, finally its automatic but living and conscious habit, the self-existent turn to do all action as a sacrifice to the Supreme and to the veiled Power present in us and in all beings and in all the workings of the universe. Life is the altar of this sacrifice, works are our offering; a transcendent and universal Power and Presence as yet rather felt or glimpsed than known or seen by us is the Deity to whom they are offered. This sacrifice, this self-consecration has two sides to it; there is the work itself and there is the spirit in which it is done, the spirit of worship to the Master of Works in all that we see, think and experience.

The work itself is at first determined by the best light we can command in our ignorance. It is that which we conceive as the thing that should be done. And whether it be shaped by our sense of duty, by our feeling for our fellow-creatures, by our idea of what is for the good of others or the good of the world or by the direction of one whom we accept as a human Master, wiser than ourselves and for us the representative of that Lord of all works in whom we believe but whom we do not yet know, the principle is the same. The essential of the sacrifice of works must be there and the essential is the surrender of all desire for the fruit of our works, the renunciation of all attachment to the result for which yet we labour. For so long as we work with attachment to the result, the sacrifice is offered not to the Divine, but to our ego.

We may think otherwise, but we are deceiving ourselves; we are making our idea of the Divine, our sense of duty, our feeling for our fellow-creatures, our idea of what is good for the world or others, even our obedience to the Master a mask for our egoistic satisfactions and preferences and a specious shield against the demand made on us to root all desire out of our nature.

At this stage of the Yoga and even throughout the Yoga this form of desire, this figure of the ego is the enemy against whom we have to be always on our guard with an unsleeping vigilance. We need not be discouraged when we find him lurking within us and assuming all sorts of disguises, but we should be vigilant to detect him in all his masks and inexorable in expelling his influence. The illumining Word of this movement is the decisive line of the Gita, "To action thou hast a right but never under any circumstances to its fruit." The fruit belongs solely to the Lord of all works; our only business with it is to prepare success by a true and careful action and to offer it, if it comes, to the divine Master. Afterwards even as we have renounced attachment to the fruit, we must renounce attachment to the work also; at any moment we must be prepared to change one work, one course or one field of action for another or abandon all works if that is the clear command of the Master. Otherwise we do the act not for his sake but for our satisfaction and pleasure in the work, from the kinetic nature's need of action or for the fulfilment of our propensities; but these are all stations and refuges of the ego. However necessary for our ordinary motion of life, they have to be abandoned in the growth of the spiritual consciousness and replaced by divine counterparts: an Ananda, an impersonal and God-directed delight will cast out or supplant the unillumined vital satisfaction and pleasure, a joyful driving of the Divine Energy the kinetic need; the fulfilment of the propensities will no longer be an object or a necessity, there will be instead the fulfilment of the Divine Will through the natural dynamic truth in action of a free soul and a luminous nature. In the end, as the attachment to the fruit of the work and to the work itself has been excised from the heart, so also the last clinging attachment to the idea and sense of ourselves as the doer has to be relinquished; the Divine Shakti must be known and felt above and within us as the true and sole worker.

∼

The renunciation of attachment to the work and its fruit is the beginning of a wide movement towards an absolute equality in the mind and soul which must become all-enveloping if we are to be perfect in the spirit. For the worship of the Master of works demands a clear recognition and glad acknowledgment of him in ourselves, in all things and in all happenings. Equality is the sign of this adoration; it is the soul's ground on which true sacrifice and worship can be done. The Lord is there equally in all beings, we have to make no essential distinctions between ourselves and others, the wise and the ignorant, friend and enemy, man and animal, the saint and the sinner. We must hate none, despise none, be repelled by none; for in all we have to see the One disguised or manifested at his pleasure. He is a little revealed in one or more revealed in another or concealed and wholly distorted in others according to his will and his knowledge of what is best for that which he intends to become in form in them and to do in works in their nature. All is ourself, one self that has taken many shapes. Hatred and disliking and scorn and repulsion, clinging and attachment and preference are natural, necessary, inevitable at a certain stage: they attend upon or they help to make and maintain Nature's choice in us. But to the Karmayogin they are a survival, a stumbling-block, a process of the Ignorance and, as he progresses, they fall away from his nature. The child-soul needs them for its growth; but they drop from an adult in the divine culture. In the God-nature to which we have to rise there can be an adamantine, even a destructive severity but not hatred, a divine irony but not scorn, a calm, clear-seeing and forceful rejection but not repulsion and dislike. Even what we have to destroy, we must not abhor or fail to recognise as a disguised and temporary movement of the Eternal.

And since all things are the one Self in its manifestation, we shall have equality of soul towards the ugly and the beautiful, the maimed and the perfect, the noble and the vulgar, the pleasant and the unpleasant, the good and the evil. Here also there will be no hatred, scorn and repulsion, but instead the equal eye that sees all things in their real character and their appointed place. For we shall know that all things express or disguise, develop or distort, as best they can or with whatever defect they must, under the circumstances intended for them, in the way possible to the immediate status or function or evolution of their nature, some truth or fact, some energy or potential of the Divine necessary by its presence in the progressive manifestation both to the whole of the present sum of things and for the perfection of the ultimate result. That truth is what we must seek and discover behind the transitory expression; undeterred by appearances, by the deficiencies or the disfigurements of the expression, we can then worship the Divine for ever unsullied, pure, beautiful and perfect behind his masks. All indeed has to be changed, not ugliness accepted but divine beauty, not imperfection taken as our resting-place but perfection striven after, the supreme good made the universal aim and not evil. But what we do has to be done with a spiritual understanding and knowledge, and it is a divine good, beauty, perfection, pleasure that has to be followed after, not the human standards of these things. If we have not equality, it is a sign that we are still pursued by the Ignorance, we shall truly understand nothing and it is more than likely that we shall destroy the old imperfection only to create another: for we are substituting the appreciations of our human mind and desire-soul for the divine values.

Equality does not mean a fresh ignorance or blindness; it does not call for and need not initiate a greyness of vision and a blotting out of all hues. Difference is there, variation of expression is there and this variation we shall appreciate,—far more justly than we could when the eye was clouded by a partial and erring love and hate, admiration and scorn, sympathy and antipathy, attraction and repulsion. But behind the variation we shall always see the Complete and Immutable who dwells within it and we shall feel, know or at least, if it is hidden from us, trust in the wise purpose and divine necessity of the particular manifestation, whether it appear to our human standards harmonious and perfect or crude and unfinished or even false and evil.

And so too we shall have the same equality of mind and soul towards all happenings, painful or pleasurable, defeat and success, honour and disgrace, good repute and ill-repute, good fortune and evil fortune. For in all happenings we shall see the will of the Master of all works and results and a step in the evolving expression of the Divine. He manifests himself, to those who have the inner eye that sees, in forces and their play and results as well as in things and in creatures. All things move towards a divine event; each experience, suffering and want no less than joy and satisfaction, is a necessary link in the carrying out of a universal movement which it is our business to understand and second. To revolt, to condemn, to cry out is the impulse of our unchastened and ignorant instincts. Revolt like everything else has its uses in the play and is even necessary, helpful, decreed for the divine development in its own time and stage; but the movement of an ignorant rebellion belongs to the stage of the soul's childhood or to its raw adolescence. The ripened soul does not condemn but seeks to understand and master, does not cry out but accepts or toils to improve and perfect, does not revolt inwardly but labours to obey and fulfil and transfigure. Therefore we shall receive all things with an equal soul from the hands of the Master. Failure we shall admit as a passage as calmly as success until the hour of the divine victory arrives. Our souls and minds and bodies will remain unshaken by acutest sorrow and suffering and pain if in the divine dispensation they come to us, unoverpowered by intensest joy and pleasure. Thus supremely balanced we shall continue steadily on our way meeting all things with an equal calm until we are ready for a more exalted status and can enter into the supreme and universal Ananda.

~

This equality cannot come except by a protracted ordeal and patient self-discipline; so long as desire is strong, equality cannot come at all except in periods of quiescence and the fatigue of desire, and it is then more likely to be an inert indifference or desire's recoil from itself than the true calm and the positive spiritual oneness. Moreover, this discipline or this growth into equality of spirit has its necessary epochs and stages. Ordinarily we have to begin with a period of endurance; for we must learn to confront, to suffer and to assimilate all contacts. Each fibre in us must be taught not to wince away from that which pains and repels and not to run eagerly towards that which pleases and attracts, but rather to accept, to face, to bear and to conquer. All touches we must be strong to bear, not only those that are proper and personal to us but those born of our sympathy or our conflict with the worlds around, above or below us and with their peoples. We shall endure tranquilly the action and impact on us of men and things and forces, the pressure of the Gods and the assaults of Titans; we shall face and engulf in the unstirred seas of our spirit all that can possibly come to us down the ways of the soul's infinite experience. This is the stoical period of the preparation of equality, its most elementary and yet its heroic age. But this steadfast endurance of the flesh and heart and mind must be reinforced by a sustained sense of spiritual submission to a divine Will: this living clay must yield not only with a stern or courageous acquiescence, but with knowledge or with resignation, even in suffering, to the touch of the divine Hand that is preparing its perfection. A sage, a devout or even a tender stoicism of the God-lover is possible, and these are better than the merely pagan self-reliant endurance which may lend itself to a too great hardening of the vessel of God: for this kind prepares the strength that is capable of wisdom and of love; its tranquillity is a deeply moved calm that passes easily into bliss. The gain of this period of resignation and endurance is the soul's strength equal to all shocks and contacts.

There is next a period of high-seated impartiality and indifference in which the soul becomes free from exultation and depression and escapes from the snare of the eagerness of joy as from the dark net of the pangs of grief and suffering. All things and persons and forces, all thoughts and feelings and sensations and actions, one's own no less than those of others, are regarded from above by a spirit that remains intact and immutable and is not disturbed by these things. This is the philosophic period of the preparation of equality, a wide and august movement. But indifference must not settle into an inert turning away from action and experience; it must not be an aversion born of weariness, disgust and distaste, a recoil of disappointed or satiated desire, the sullenness of a baffled and dissatisfied egoism forced back from its passionate aims. These recoils come inevitably in the unripe soul and may in some way help the progress by a discouragement of the eager desire-driven vital nature, but they are not the perfection towards which we labour. The indifference or the impartiality that we must seek after is a calm superiority of the high-seated soul above the contacts of things;[1] it regards and accepts or rejects them but is not moved in the rejection and is not subjected by the acceptance. It begins to feel itself near, kin to, one with a silent Self and Spirit self-existent and separate from the workings of Nature which it supports and makes possible, part of or merged in the motionless calm Reality that transcends the motion and action of the universe. The gain of this period of high transcendence is the soul's peace unrocked and unshaken by the pleasant ripplings or by the tempestuous waves and billows of the world's movement.

If we can pass through these two stages of the inner change without being arrested or fixed in either, we are admitted to a greater divine equality which is capable of a spiritual ardour and tranquil passion of delight, a rapturous, all-understanding and all-possessing equality of the perfected soul, an intense and even wideness and fullness of its being embracing all things. This is the supreme period and the passage to it is through the joy of a total self-giving to the Divine and to the universal Mother. For strength is then crowned by a happy mastery, peace deepens into bliss, the possession of the divine calm is uplifted and made the ground for the possession of the divine movement. But if this greater perfection is to arrive, the soul's impartial high-seatedness looking down from above on the flux of forms and personalities and movements and forces must be modified and change into a new sense of strong and calm submission and a powerful and intense surrender. This submission will be no longer a resigned acquiescence but a glad acceptance: for there will be no sense of suffering or of the bearing of a burden or cross; love and delight and the joy of self-giving will be its brilliant texture. And this surrender will be not only to a divine Will which we perceive and accept and obey, but to a divine Wisdom in the Will which we recognise and a divine Love in it which we feel and rapturously suffer, the wisdom and love of a supreme Spirit and Self of ourselves and all with which we can achieve a happy and perfect unity. A lonely power, peace and stillness is the last word of the philosophic equality of the sage; but the soul in its integral experience liberates itself from this self-created status and enters into the sea of a supreme and all-embracing ecstasy of the beginningless and endless beatitude of the Eternal. Then we are at last capable of receiving all contacts with a blissful equality, because we feel in them the touch of the imperishable Love and Delight, the happiness absolute that hides ever in the heart of things. The gain of this culmination in a universal and equal rapture is the soul's delight and the opening gates of the Bliss that is infinite, the Joy that surpasses all understanding.

Before this labour for the annihilation of desire and the conquest of the soul's equality can come to its absolute perfection and fruition, that turn of the spiritual movement must have been completed which leads to the abolition of the sense of ego. But for the worker the renunciation of the egoism of action is the most important element in this change. For even when by giving up the fruits and the desire of the fruits to the Master of the Sacrifice we have parted with the egoism of rajasic desire, we may still have kept the egoism of the worker. Still we are subject to the sense that we are ourselves the doer of the act, ourselves its source and ourselves the giver of the sanction. It is still the "I" that chooses and determines, it is still the "I" that undertakes the responsibility and feels the demerit or the merit.

An entire removal of this separative ego-sense is an essential aim of our Yoga. If any ego is to remain in us for a while, it is only a form of it which knows itself to be a form and is ready to disappear as soon as a true centre of consciousness is manifested or built in us. That true centre is a luminous formulation of the one Consciousness and a pure channel and instrument of the one Existence. A support for the individual manifestation and action of the universal Force, it gradually reveals behind it the true Person in us, the central eternal being, an everlasting being of the Supreme, a power and portion of the transcendent Shakti.[2]

Here too, in this movement by which the soul divests itself gradually of the obscure robe of the ego, there is a progress by marked stages. For not only the fruit of works belongs to the Lord alone, but our works also must be his; he is the true lord of our actions no less than of our results. This we must not see with the thinking mind only, it must become entirely true to our entire consciousness and will. The sadhaka has not only to think and know but to see and feel concretely and intensely even in the moment of the working and in its initiation and whole process that his works are not his at all, but are coming through him from the Supreme Existence. He must be always aware of a Force, a Presence, a Will that acts through his individual nature. But there is in taking this turn the danger that he may confuse his own disguised or sublimated ego or an inferior power with the Lord and substitute its demands for the supreme dictates. He may fall into a common ambush of this lower nature and distort his supposed surrender to a higher Power into an excuse for a magnified and uncontrolled indulgence of his own self-will and even of his desires and passions. A great sincerity is asked for and has to be imposed not only on the conscious mind but still more on the subliminal part of us which is full of hidden movements. For there is there, especially in our subliminal vital nature, an incorrigible charlatan and actor. The sadhaka must first have advanced far in the elimination of desire and in the firm equality of his soul towards all workings and all happenings before he can utterly lay down the burden of his works on the Divine. At every moment he must proceed with a vigilant eye upon the deceits of the ego and the ambushes of the misleading Powers of Darkness who ever represent themselves as the one Source of Light and Truth and take on them a simulacrum of divine forms in order to capture the soul of the seeker.

Immediately he must take the further step of relegating himself to the position of the Witness. Aloof from the Prakriti, impersonal and dispassionate, he must watch the executive Nature-Force at work within him and understand its action; he must learn by this separation to recognise the play of her universal forces, distinguish her interweaving of light and night, the divine and the undivine, and detect her formidable Powers and Beings that use the ignorant human creature. Nature works in us, says the Gita, through the triple quality of Prakriti, the quality of light and good, the quality of passion and desire and the quality of obscurity and inertia. The seeker must learn to distinguish, as an impartial and discerning witness of all that proceeds within this kingdom of his nature, the separate and the combined action of these qualities; he must pursue the workings of the cosmic forces in him through all the labyrinth of their subtle unseen processes and disguises and know every intricacy of the maze. As he proceeds in this knowledge, he will be able to become the giver of the sanction and no longer remain an ignorant tool of Nature. At first he must induce the NatureForce in its action on his instruments to subdue the working of its two lower qualities and bring them into subjection to the quality of light and good and, afterwards, he must persuade that again to offer itself so that all three may be transformed by a higher Power into their divine equivalents, supreme repose and calm, divine illumination and bliss, the eternal divine dynamis, Tapas. The first part of this discipline and change can be firmly done in principle by the will of the mental being in us; but its full execution and the subsequent transformation can be done only when the deeper psychic soul increases its hold on the nature and replaces the mental being as its ruler. When this happens, he will be ready to make, not only with an aspiration and intention and an initial and progressive self-abandonment but with the most intense actuality of dynamic self-giving, the complete renunciation of his works to the Supreme Will. By degrees his mind of an imperfect human intelligence will be replaced by a spiritual and illumined mind and that can in the end enter into the supramental Truth-Light; he will then no longer act from his nature of the Ignorance with its three modes of confused and imperfect activity, but from a diviner nature of spiritual calm, light, power and bliss. He will act not from an amalgam of an ignorant mind and will with the drive of a still more ignorant heart of emotion and the desire of the life-being and the urge and instinct of the flesh, but first from a spiritualised self and nature and, last, from a supramental Truth-consciousness and its divine force of supernature.

Thus are made possible the final steps when the veil of Nature is withdrawn and the seeker is face to face with the Master of all existence and his activities are merged in the action of a supreme Energy which is pure, true, perfect and blissful for ever. Thus can he utterly renounce to the supramental Shakti his works as well as the fruits of his works and act only as the conscious instrument of the eternal Worker. No longer giving the sanction, he will rather receive in his instruments and follow in her hands divine mandate. No longer doing works, he will accept their execution through him by her unsleeping Force. No longer willing the fulfilment of his own mental constructions and the satisfaction of his own emotional desires, he will obey and participate in an omnipotent Will that is also an omniscient Knowledge and a mysterious, magical and unfathomable Love and a vast bottomless sea of the eternal Bliss of Existence.

---

1. *udāsīna*.
2. *aṁśaḥ sanātanaḥ, parā prakṛtir jīvabhūta*.

CHAPTER X. THE THREE MODES OF NATURE

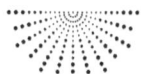

TO TRANSCEND the natural action of the lower Prakriti is indispensable to the soul, if it is to be free in its self and free in its works. Harmonious subjection to this actual universal Nature, a condition of good and perfect work for the natural instruments, is not an ideal for the soul, which should rather be subject to God and his Shakti, but master of its own nature. As agent or as channel of the Supreme Will it must determine by its vision and sanction or refusal the use that shall be made of the storage of energy, the conditions of environment, the rhythm of combined movement which are provided by Prakriti for the labour of the natural instruments, mind, life and body. But this inferior Nature can only be mastered if she is surmounted and used from above. And this can only be done by a transcendence of her forces, qualities and modes of action; otherwise we are subject to her conditions and helplessly dominated by her, not free in the spirit.

The idea of the three essential modes of Nature is a creation of the ancient Indian thinkers and its truth is not at once obvious, because it was the result of long psychological experiment and profound internal experience. Therefore without a long inner experience, without intimate self-observation and intuitive perception of the Nature-forces it is difficult to grasp accurately or firmly utilise. Still certain broad indications may help the seeker on the Way of Works to understand, analyse and control by his assent or refusal the combinations of his own nature. These modes are termed in the Indian books qualities, *guṇas*, and are given the names *sattva, rajas, tamas*. Sattwa is the force of equilibrium and translates in quality as good and harmony and happiness and light; rajas is the force of kinesis and translates in quality as struggle and effort, passion and action; tamas is the force of inconscience and inertia and translates in quality as obscurity and incapacity and inaction. Ordinarily used for psychological self-analysis, these distinctions are valid also in physical Nature. Each thing and every existence in the lower Prakriti contains them and its process and dynamic form are the result of the interaction of these qualitative powers.

Every form of things, whether animate or inanimate, is a constantly maintained poise of natural forces in motion and is subject to an unending stream of helpful, disturbing or disintegrating contacts from other combinations of forces that surround it. Our own nature of mind, life and body is nothing else than such a formative combination and poise. In the reception of the environing contacts and the reaction to them the three modes determine the temper of the recipient and the character of the response. Inert and inapt, he may suffer them without any responsive reaction, any motion of self-defence or any capacity of assimilation and adjustment; this is the mode of tamas, the way of inertia. The stigmata of tamas are blindness and unconsciousness and incapacity and unintelligence, sloth and indolence and inactivity and mechanical routine and the mind's torpor and the life's sleep and the soul's slumber. Its effect, if uncorrected by other elements, can be nothing but disintegration of the form or the poise of the nature without any new creation or new equilibrium or force of kinetic progress. At the heart of this inert impotence is the principle of ignorance and an inability or slothful unwillingness to comprehend, seize and manage the stimulating or assailing contact, the suggestion of environing forces and their urge towards fresh experience.

On the other hand, the recipient of Nature's contacts, touched and stimulated, solicited or assailed by her forces, may react to the pressure or against it. She allows, encourages, impels him to strive, to resist, to attempt, to dominate or engross his environment, to assert his will, to fight and create and conquer. This is the mode of rajas, the way of passion and action and the thirst of desire. Struggle and change and new creation, victory and defeat and joy and suffering and hope and disappointment are its children and build the many-coloured house of life in which it takes its pleasure. But its knowledge is an imperfect or a false knowledge and brings with it ignorant effort, error, a constant misadjustment, pain of attachment, disappointed desire, grief of loss and failure. The gift of rajas is kinetic force, energy, activity, the power that creates and acts and can overcome; but it moves in the wrong lights or the half-lights of the Ignorance and it is perverted by the touch of the Asura, Rakshasa and Pishacha. The arrogant ignorance of the human mind and its self-satisfied perversions and presumptuous errors, the pride and vanity and ambition, the cruelty and tyranny and beast wrath and violence, the selfishness and baseness and hypocrisy and treachery and vile meanness, the lust and greed and rapacity, the jealousy, envy and bottomless ingratitude that disfigure the earth-nature are the natural children of this indispensable but strong and dangerous turn of Nature.

But the embodied being is not limited to these two modes of Prakriti; there is a better and more enlightened way in which he can deal with surrounding impacts and the stream of the world-forces. There is possible a reception and reaction with clear comprehension, poise and balance. This way of natural being has the power that, because it understands, sympathises; it fathoms and controls and develops Nature's urge and her ways: it has an intelligence that penetrates her processes and her significances and can assimilate and utilise; there is a lucid response that is not overpowered but adjusts, corrects, adapts, harmonises, elicits the best in all things. This is the mode of sattwa, the turn of Nature that is full of light and poise, directed to good, to knowledge, to delight and beauty, to happiness, right understanding, right equilibrium, right order: its temperament is the opulence of a bright clearness of knowledge and a lucent warmth of sympathy and closeness. A fineness and enlightenment, a governed energy, an accomplished harmony and poise of the whole being is the consummate achievement of the sattwic nature.

No existence is cast entirely in the single mould of any of these three modes of the cosmic Force; all three are present in everyone and everywhere. There is a constant combining and separation of their shifting relations and interpenetrating influences, often a conflict, a wrestling of forces, a struggle to dominate each other. All have in great or in small extent or degree, even if sometimes in a hardly appreciable minimum, their sattwic states and clear tracts or inchoate tendencies of light, clarity and happiness, fine adaptation and sympathy with the environment, intelligence, poise, right mind, right will and feeling, right impulse, virtue, order. All have their rajasic moods and impulses and turbid parts of desire and passion and struggle, perversion and falsehood and error, unbalanced joy and sorrow, aggressive push to work and eager creation and strong or bold or fiery or fierce reactions to the pressure of the environment and to life's assaults and offers. All have their tamasic states and constant obscure parts, their moments or points of unconsciousness, their long habit or their temporary velleities of weak resignation or dull acceptance, their constitutional feeblenesses or movements of fatigue, negligence and indolence and their lapses into ignorance and incapacity, depression and fear and cowardly recoil or submission to the environment and to the pressure of men and events and forces. Each one of us is sattwic in some directions of his energy of Nature or in some parts of his mind or character, in others rajasic, tamasic in others. According as one or other of the modes usually dominates his general temperament and type of mind and turn of action, it is said of him that he is the sattwic, the rajasic or the tamasic man; but few are always of one kind and none is entire in his kind. The wise are not always or wholly wise, the intelligent are intelligent only in patches; the saint suppresses in himself many unsaintly movements and the evil are not entirely evil: the dullest has his unexpressed or unused and undeveloped capacities, the most timorous his moments or his way of courage, the helpless and the weakling a latent part of strength in his nature. The dominant gunas are not the essential soul-type of the embodied being but only the index of the formation he has made for this life or during his present existence and at a given moment of his evolution in Time.

∼

When the sadhaka has once stood back from the action of Prakriti within him or upon him and, not interfering, not amending or inhibiting, not choosing or deciding, allowed its play and analysed and watched the process, he soon discovers that her modes are self-dependent and work as a machine once put in action works by its own structure and propelling forces. The force and the propulsion come from Prakriti and not from the creature. Then he realises how mistaken was his impression that his mind was the doer of his works; his mind was only a small part of him and a creation and engine of Nature. Nature was acting all the while in her own modes moving the three general qualities about as a girl might play with her puppets. His ego was all along a tool and plaything; his character and intelligence, his moral qualities and mental powers, his creations and works and exploits, his anger and forbearance, his cruelty and mercy, his love and his hatred, his sin and his virtue, his light and his darkness, his passion of joy and his anguish of sorrow were the play of Nature to which the soul, attracted, won and subjected, lent its passive concurrence. And yet the determinism of Nature or Force is not all; the soul has a word to say in the matter,—but the secret soul, the Purusha, not the mind or the ego, since these are not independent entities, they are parts of Nature. For the soul's sanction is needed for the play and by an inner silent will as the lord and giver of the sanction it can determine the principle of the play and intervene in its combinations, although the execution in thought and will and act and impulse must still be Nature's part and privilege. The Purusha can dictate a harmony for Nature to execute, not by interfering in her functions but by a conscious regard on her which she transmutes at once or after much difficulty into translating idea and dynamic impetus and significant figure.

An escape from the action of the two inferior gunas is very evidently indispensable if we are to transmute our present nature into a power and form of the divine consciousness and an instrument of its forces. Tamas obscures and prevents the light of the divine knowledge from penetrating into the dark and dull corners of our nature. Tamas incapacitates and takes away the power to respond to divine impulse and the energy to change and the will to progress and make ourselves plastic to a greater Shakti.

Rajas perverts knowledge, makes our reason the accomplice of falsehood and the abettor of every wrong movement, disturbs and twists our life-force and its impulses, oversets the balance and health of the body. Rajas captures all high-born ideas and high-seated movements and turns them to a false and egoistic use; even divine Truth and divine influences, when they descend into the earthly plane, cannot escape this misuse and seizure. Tamas unenlightened and rajas unconverted, no divine change or divine life is possible.

An exclusive resort to sattwa would seem to be the way of escape: but there is this difficulty that no one of the qualities can prevail by itself against its two companions and rivals. If, envisaging the quality of desire and passion as the cause of disturbance, suffering, sin and sorrow, we strain and labour to quell and subdue it, rajas sinks but tamas rises. For, the principle of activity dulled, inertia takes its place. A quiet peace, happiness, knowledge, love, right sentiment can be founded by the principle of light, but, if rajas is absent or completely suppressed, the quiet in the soul tends to become a tranquillity of inaction, not the firm ground of a dynamic change. Ineffectively right-thinking, right-doing, good, mild and even, the nature may become in its dynamic parts sattwa-tamasic, neutral, pale-tinted, uncreative or emptied of power. Mental and moral obscurity may be absent, but so are the intense springs of action, and this is a hampering limitation and another kind of incompetence. For tamas is a double principle; it contradicts rajas by inertia, it contradicts sattwa by narrowness, obscurity and ignorance and, if either is depressed, it pours in to occupy its place.

If we call in rajas again to correct this error and bid it ally itself to sattwa and by their united agency endeavour to get rid of the dark principle, we find that we have elevated our action, but that there is again subjection to rajasic eagerness, passion, disappointment, suffering, anger. These movements may be more exalted in their scope and spirit and action than before, but they are not the peace, the freedom, the power, the self-mastery at which we long to arrive. Wherever desire and ego harbour, passion and disturbance harbour with them and share their life. And if we seek a compromise between the three modes, sattwa leading, the others subordinate, still we have only arrived at a more temperate action of the play of Nature. A new poise has been reached, but a spiritual freedom and mastery are not in sight or else are still only a far-off prospect.

A radically different movement has to draw us back from the gunas and lift us above them. The error that accepts the action of the modes of Nature must cease; for as long as it is accepted, the soul is involved in their operations and subjected to their law. Sattwa must be transcended as well as rajas and tamas; the golden chain must be broken no less than the leaden fetters and the bond-ornaments of a mixed alloy. The Gita prescribes to this end a new method of self-discipline. It is to stand back in oneself from the action of the modes and observe this unsteady flux as the Witness seated above the surge of the forces of Nature. He is one who watches but is impartial and indifferent, aloof from them on their own level and in his native posture high above them. As they rise and fall in their waves, the Witness looks, observes, but neither accepts nor for the moment interferes with their course. First there must be the freedom of the impersonal Witness; afterwards there can be the control of the Master, the Ishwara.

~

The initial advantage of this process of detachment is that one begins to understand one's own nature and all Nature. The detached Witness is able to see entirely without the least blinding by egoism the play of her modes of the Ignorance and to pursue it into all its ramifications, coverings and subtleties—for it is full of camouflage and disguise and snare and treachery and ruse. Instructed by long experience, conscious of all act and condition as their interaction, made wise of their processes, he cannot any longer be overcome by their assaults, surprised in their nets or deceived by their disguises. At the same time he perceives the ego to be nothing better than a device and the sustaining knot of their interaction and, perceiving it, he is delivered from the illusion of the lower egoistic Nature. He escapes from the sattwic egoism of the altruist and the saint and the thinker; he shakes off from its control on his life-impulses the rajasic egoism of the self-seeker and ceases to be the laborious caterer of self-interest and the pampered prisoner or toiling galley-slave of passion and desire; he slays with the light of knowledge the tamasic egoism of the ignorant or passive being, dull, unintelligent, attached to the common round of human life. Thus convinced and conscious of the essential vice of the ego-sense in all our personal action, he seeks no longer to find a means of self-correction and self-liberation in the rajasic or sattwic ego but looks above, beyond the instruments and the working of Nature, to the Master of works alone and his supreme Shakti, the supreme Prakriti. There alone all the being is pure and free and the rule of a divine Truth possible.

In this progression the first step is a certain detached superiority to the three modes of Nature. The soul is inwardly separated and free from the lower Prakriti, not involved in its coils, indifferent and glad above it. Nature continues to act in the triple round of her ancient habits,—desire, grief and joy attack the heart, the instruments fall into inaction and obscurity and weariness, light and peace come back into the heart and mind and body; but the soul stands unchanged and untouched by these changes. Observing and unmoved by the grief and desire of the lower members, smiling at their joys and their strainings, regarding and unoverpowered by the failing and the darknesses of the thought and the wildness or the weaknesses of the heart and nerves, uncompelled and unattached to the mind's illuminations and its relief and sense of ease or of power in the return of light and gladness, it throws itself into none of these things, but waits unmoved for the intimations of a higher Will and the intuitions of a greater luminous knowledge. Thus doing always, it becomes eventually free even in its nature parts from the strife of the three modes and their insufficient values and imprisoning limits. For now this lower Prakriti feels progressively a compulsion from a higher Shakti. The old habits to which it clung receive no further sanction and begin steadily to lose their frequency and force of recurrence. At last it understands that it is called to a higher action and a better state and, however slowly, however reluctantly, with whatever initial or prolonged ill-will and stumbling ignorance, it submits, turns and prepares itself for the change.

The static freedom of the soul, no longer witness only and knower, is crowned by a dynamic transformation of the nature. The constant mixture, the uneven operation of the three modes acting upon each other in our three instruments ceases from its normal confused, troubled and improper action and movement. Another action becomes possible, commences, grows, culminates, a working more truly right, more luminous, natural and normal to the deepest divine interplay of Purusha and Prakriti although supernatural and supernormal to our present imperfect nature. The body conditioning the physical mind insists no longer on its tamasic inertia that repeats always the same ignorant movement: it becomes a passive field and instrument of a greater force and light, it responds to every demand of the spirit's force, holds and supports every variety and intensity of new divine experience. Our kinetic and dynamic vital parts, our nervous and emotional and sensational and volitional being, expand in power and admit a tireless action and a blissful enjoyment of experience, but learn at the same time to stand on a foundation of wide self-possessed and self-poised calm, sublime in force, divine in rest, neither exulting and excited nor tortured by sorrow and pain, neither harried by desire and importunate impulses nor dulled by incapacity and indolence. The intelligence, the thinking, understanding and reflective mind, renounces its sattwic limitations and opens to an essential light and peace. An infinite knowledge offers to us its splendid ranges, a knowledge not made up of mental constructions, not bound by opinion and idea or dependent on a stumbling uncertain logic and the petty support of the senses, but self-sure, authentic, all-penetrating, all-comprehending; a boundless bliss and peace, not dependent on deliverance from the hampered strenuousness of creative energy and dynamic action, not constituted by a few limited felicities but self-existent and all-including, pour into ever-enlarging fields and through ever-widening and always more numerous channels to possess the nature. A higher force, bliss and knowledge from a source beyond mind and life and body seize on them to remould in a diviner image.

Here the disharmonies of the triple mode of our inferior existence are overpassed and there begins a greater triple mode of a divine Nature. There is no obscurity of tamas or inertia. Tamas is replaced by a divine peace and tranquil eternal repose out of which is released from a supreme matrix of calm concentration the play of action and knowledge. There is no rajasic kinesis, no desire, no joyful and sorrowful striving of action, creation and possession, no fruitful chaos of troubled impulse. Rajas is replaced by a self-possessed power and illimitable act of force, that even in its most violent intensities does not shake the immovable poise of the soul or stain the vast and profound heavens and luminous abysses of its peace. There is no constructing light of mind casting about to seize and imprison the Truth, no insecure or inactive ease. Sattwa is replaced by an illumination and a spiritual bliss identical with the depth and infinite existence of the soul and instinct with a direct and authentic knowledge that springs straight from the veiled glories of the secret Omniscience.

This is the greater consciousness into which our inferior consciousness has to be transformed, this nature of the Ignorance with its unquiet unbalanced activity of the three modes changed into this greater luminous supernature. At first we become free from the three gunas, detached, untroubled, *nistraiguṇya*; but this is the recovery of the native state of the soul, the self, the spirit free and watching in its motionless calm the motion of Prakriti in her force of the Ignorance. If on this basis the nature, the motion of Prakriti, is also to become free, it must be by a quiescence of action in a luminous peace and silence in which all necessary movements are done without any conscious reaction or participation or initiation of action by the mind or by the lifebeing, without any ripple of thought or eddy of the vital parts: it must be done under the impulsion, by the initiation, by the working of an impersonal cosmic or a transcendent Force. A cosmic Mind, Life, Substance must act, or a pure transcendent Self-Power and Bliss other than our own personal being or its building of Nature. This is a state of freedom which can come in the Yoga of works through renunciation of ego and desire and personal initiation and the surrender of the being to the cosmic Self or to the universal Shakti; it can come in the Yoga of knowledge by the cessation of thought, the silence of the mind, the opening of the whole being to the cosmic Consciousness, to the cosmic Self, the cosmic Dynamis or to the supreme Reality; it can come in the Yoga of devotion by the surrender of the heart and the whole nature into the hands of the All-Blissful as the adored Master of our existence. But the culminating change intervenes by a more positive and dynamic transcendence: there is a transference or transmutation into a superior spiritual status, *triguṇātīta*, in which we participate in a greater spiritual dynamisation; for the three lower unequal modes pass into an equal triune mode of eternal calm, light and force, the repose, kinesis, illumination of the divine Nature.

This supreme harmony cannot come except by the cessation of egoistic will and choice and act and the quiescence of our limited intelligence. The individual ego must cease to strive, the mind fall silent, the desire-will learn not to initiate. Our personality must join its source and all thought and initiation come from above. The secret Master of our activities will be slowly unveiled to us and from the security of the supreme Will and Knowledge give the sanction to the Divine Shakti who will do all works in us with a purified and exalted nature for her instrument; the individual centre of personality will be only the upholder of her works here, their recipient and channel, the reflector of her power and luminous participator in her light, joy and force. Acting it will not act and no reaction of the lower Prakriti will touch it. The transcendence of the three modes of Nature is the first condition, their transformation the decisive step of this change by which the Way of Works climbs out of the pit of narrowness of our darkened human nature into the unwalled wideness of the Truth and Light above us.

CHAPTER XI. THE MASTER OF THE WORK

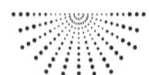

THE MASTER and Mover of our works is the One, the Universal and Supreme, the Eternal and Infinite. He is the transcendent unknown or unknowable Absolute, the unexpressed and unmanifested Ineffable above us; but he is also the Self of all beings, the Master of all worlds, transcending all worlds, the Light and the Guide, the All-Beautiful and AllBlissful, the Beloved and the Lover. He is the Cosmic Spirit and all-creating Energy around us; he is the Immanent within us. All that is is he, and he is the More than all that is, and we ourselves, though we know it not, are being of his being, force of his force, conscious with a consciousness derived from his; even our mortal existence is made out of his substance and there is an immortal within us that is a spark of the Light and Bliss that are for ever. No matter whether by knowledge, works, love or any other means, to become aware of this truth of our being, to realise it, to make it effective here or elsewhere is the object of all Yoga.

But the passage is long and the labour arduous before we can look on him with eyes that see true, and still longer and more arduous must be our endeavour if we would rebuild ourselves in his true image. The Master of the work does not reveal himself at once to the seeker. Always it is his Power that acts behind the veil, but it is manifest only when we renounce the egoism of the worker, and its direct movement increases in proportion as that renunciation becomes more and more complete. Only when our surrender to his Divine Shakti is absolute, shall we have the right to live in his absolute presence. And only then can we see our work throw itself naturally, completely and simply into the mould of the Divine Will.

There must, therefore, be stages and gradations in our approach to this perfection, as there are in the progress towards all other perfection on any plane of Nature. The vision of the full glory may come to us before, suddenly or slowly, once or often, but until the foundation is complete, it is a summary and concentrated, not a durable and all-enveloping experience, not a lasting presence. The amplitudes, the infinite contents of the Divine Revelation come afterwards and unroll gradually their power and their significance. Or, even, the steady vision can be there on the summits of our nature, but the perfect response of the lower members comes only by degrees. In all Yoga the first requisites are faith and patience. The ardours of the heart and the violences of the eager will that seek to take the kingdom of heaven by storm can have miserable reactions if they disdain to support their vehemence on these humbler and quieter auxiliaries. And in the long and difficult integral Yoga there must be an integral faith and an unshakable patience.

It is difficult to acquire or to practise this faith and steadfastness on the rough and narrow path of Yoga because of the impatience of both heart and mind and the eager but soon faltering will of our rajasic nature. The vital nature of man hungers always for the fruit of its labour and, if the fruit appears to be denied or long delayed, he loses faith in the ideal and in the guidance. For his mind judges always by the appearance of things, since that is the first ingrained habit of the intellectual reason in which he so inordinately trusts. Nothing is easier for us than to accuse God in our hearts when we suffer long or stumble in the darkness or to abjure the ideal that we have set before us. For we say, "I have trusted to the Highest and I am betrayed into suffering and sin and error." Or else, "I have staked my whole life on an idea which the stern facts of experience contradict and discourage. It would have been better to be as other men are who accept their limitations and walk on the firm ground of normal experience." In such moments—and they are sometimes frequent and long—all the higher experience is forgotten and the heart concentrates itself in its own bitterness. It is in these dark passages that it is possible to fall for good or to turn back from the divine labour.

If one has walked long and steadily in the path, the faith of the heart will remain under the fiercest adverse pressure; even if it is concealed or apparently overborne, it will take the first opportunity to re-emerge. For something higher than either heart or intellect upholds it in spite of the worst stumblings and through the most prolonged failure. But even to the experienced sadhaka such falterings or overcloudings bring a retardation of his progress and they are exceedingly dangerous to the novice. It is therefore necessary from the beginning to understand and accept the arduous difficulty of the path and to feel the need of a faith which to the intellect may seem blind, but yet is wiser than our reasoning intelligence. For this faith is a support from above; it is the brilliant shadow thrown by a secret light that exceeds the intellect and its data; it is the heart of a hidden knowledge that is not at the mercy of immediate appearances. Our faith, persevering, will be justified in its works and will be lifted and transfigured at last into the self-revelation of a divine knowledge. Always we must adhere to the injunction of the Gita, "Yoga must be continually applied with a heart free from despondent sinking." Always we must repeat to the doubting intellect the promise of the Master, "I will surely deliver thee from all sin and evil; do not grieve." At the end, the flickerings of faith will cease; for we shall see his face and feel always the Divine Presence.

The Master of our works respects our nature even when he is transforming it; he works always through the nature and not by any arbitrary caprice. This imperfect nature of ours contains the materials of our perfection, but inchoate, distorted, misplaced, thrown together in disorder or a poor imperfect order. All this material has to be patiently perfected, purified, reorganised, new-moulded and transformed, not hacked and hewn and slain or mutilated, not obliterated by simple coercion and denial. This world and we who live in it are his creation and manifestation, and he deals with it and us in a way our narrow and ignorant mind cannot understand unless it falls silent and opens to a divine knowledge. In our errors is the substance of a truth which labours to reveal its meaning to our groping intelligence. The human intellect cuts out the error and the truth with it and replaces it by another half-truth half-error; but the Divine Wisdom suffers our mistakes to continue until we are able to arrive at the truth hidden and protected under every false cover. Our sins are the misdirected steps of a seeking Power that aims, not at sin, but at perfection, at something that we might call a divine virtue. Often they are the veils of a quality that has to be transformed and delivered out of this ugly disguise: otherwise, in the perfect providence of things, they would not have been suffered to exist or to continue. The Master of our works is neither a blunderer nor an indifferent witness nor a dallier with the luxury of unneeded evils. He is wiser than our reason and wiser than our virtue.

Our nature is not only mistaken in will and ignorant in knowledge but weak in power; but the Divine Force is there and will lead us if we trust in it and it will use our deficiencies and our powers for the divine purpose. If we fail in our immediate aim, it is because he has intended the failure; often our failure or ill-result is the right road to a truer issue than an immediate and complete success would have put in our reach. If we suffer, it is because something in us has to be prepared for a rarer possibility of delight. If we stumble, it is to learn in the end the secret of a more perfect walking. Let us not be in too furious a haste to acquire even peace, purity and perfection. Peace must be ours, but not the peace of an empty or devastated nature or of slain or mutilated capacities incapable of unrest because we have made them incapable of intensity and fire and force. Purity must be our aim, but not the purity of a void or of a bleak and rigid coldness. Perfection is demanded of us, but not the perfection that can exist only by confining its scope within narrow limits or putting an arbitrary full stop to the ever self-extending scroll of the Infinite. Our object is to change into the divine nature, but the divine nature is not a mental or moral but a spiritual condition, difficult to achieve, difficult even to conceive by our intelligence. The Master of our work and our Yoga knows the thing to be done, and we must allow him to do it in us by his own means and in his own manner.

The movement of the Ignorance is egoistic at its core and nothing is more difficult for us than to get rid of egoism while yet we admit personality and adhere to action in the half-light and half-force of our unfinished nature. It is easier to starve the ego by renouncing the impulse to act or to kill it by cutting away from us all movement of personality. It is easier to exalt it into self-forgetfulness immersed in a trance of peace or an ecstasy of divine Love. But our more difficult problem is to liberate the true Person and attain to a divine manhood which shall be the pure vessel of a divine force and the perfect instrument of a divine action. Step after step has to be firmly taken; difficulty after difficulty has to be entirely experienced and entirely mastered. Only the Divine Wisdom and Power can do this for us and it will do all if we yield to it in an entire faith and follow and assent to its workings with a constant courage and patience.

The first step on this long path is to consecrate all our works as a sacrifice to the Divine in us and in the world; this is an attitude of the mind and heart, not too difficult to initiate, but very difficult to make absolutely sincere and all-pervasive. The second step is to renounce attachment to the fruit of our works; for the only true, inevitable and utterly desirable fruit of sacrifice—the one thing needful—is the Divine Presence and the Divine Consciousness and Power in us, and if that is gained, all else will be added. This is a transformation of the egoistic will in our vital being, our desire-soul and desire-nature, and it is far more difficult than the other. The third step is to get rid of the central egoism and even the ego-sense of the worker. That is the most difficult transformation of all and it cannot be perfectly done if the first two steps have not been taken; but these first steps too cannot be completed unless the third comes in to crown the movement and, by the extinction of egoism, eradicates the very origin of desire. Only when the small ego-sense is rooted out from the nature can the seeker know his true person that stands above as a portion and power of the Divine and renounce all motive-force other than the will of the Divine Shakti.

∼

There are gradations in this last integralising movement; for it cannot be done at once or without long approaches that bring it progressively nearer and make it at last possible. The first attitude to be taken is to cease to regard ourselves as the worker and firmly to realise that we are only one instrument of the cosmic Force. At first it is not the one Force but many cosmic forces that seem to move us; but these may be turned into feeders of the ego and this vision liberates the mind but not the rest of the nature. Even when we become aware of all as the working of one cosmic Force and of the Divine behind it, that too need not liberate. If the egoism of the worker disappears, the egoism of the instrument may replace it or else prolong it in a disguise. The life of the world has been full of instances of egoism of this kind and it can be more engrossing and enormous than any other; there is the same danger in Yoga. A man becomes a leader of men or eminent in a large or lesser circle and feels himself full of a power that he knows to be beyond his own ego-force; he may be aware of a Fate acting through him or a Will mysterious and unfathomable or a Light within of great brilliance. There are extraordinary results of his thoughts, his actions or his creative genius. He effects some tremendous destruction that clears the path for humanity or some great construction that becomes its momentary resting-place. He is a scourge or he is a bringer of light and healing, a creator of beauty or a messenger of knowledge. Or, if his work and its effects are on a lesser scale and have limited field, still they are attended by the strong sense that he is an instrument and chosen for his mission or his labour. Men who have this destiny and these powers come easily to believe and declare themselves to be mere instruments in the hand of God or of Fate: but even in the declaration we can see that there can intrude or take refuge an intenser and more exaggerated egoism than ordinary men have the courage to assert or the strength to house within them. And often if men of this kind speak of God, it is to erect an image of him which is really nothing but a huge shadow of themselves or their own nature, a sustaining Deific Essence of their own type of will and thought and quality and force. This magnified image of their ego is the Master whom they serve. This happens only too often in Yoga to strong but crude vital natures or minds too easily exalted when they allow ambition, pride or the desire of greatness to enter into their spiritual seeking and vitiate its purity of motive; a magnified ego stands between them and their true being and grasps for its own personal purpose the strength from a greater unseen Power, divine or undivine, acting through them of which they become vaguely or intensely aware. An intellectual perception or vital sense of a

Force greater than ours and of ourselves as moved by it is not sufficient to liberate from the ego.

This perception, this sense of a greater Power in us or above and moving us, is not a hallucination or a megalomania. Those who thus feel and see have a larger sight than ordinary men and have advanced a step beyond the limited physical intelligence, but theirs is not the plenary vision or the direct experience. For, because they are not clear in mind and aware in the soul, because their awakening is more in the vital parts than into the spiritual substance of Self, they cannot be the conscious instruments of the Divine or come face to face with the Master, but are used through their fallible and imperfect nature. The most they see of the Divinity is a Fate or a cosmic Force or else they give his name to a limited Godhead or, worse, to a Titanic or demoniac Power that veils him. Even certain religious founders have erected the image of the God of a sect or a national God or a Power of terror and punishment or a Numen of sattwic love and mercy and virtue and seem not to have seen the One and Eternal. The Divine accepts the image they make of him and does his work in them through that medium, but, since the one Force is felt and acts in their imperfect nature but more intensely than in others, the motive principle of egoism too can be more intense in them than in others. An exalted rajasic or sattwic ego still holds them and stands between them and the integral Truth. Even this is something, a beginning, although far from the true and perfect experience. A much worse thing may befall those who break something of the human bonds but have not purity and have not the knowledge, for they may become instruments, but not of the Divine; too often, using his name, they serve unconsciously his Masks and black Contraries, the Powers of Darkness.

Our nature must house the cosmic Force but not in its lower aspect or in its rajasic or sattwic movement; it must serve the universal Will, but in the light of a greater liberating knowledge. There must be no egoism of any kind in the attitude of the instrument, even when we are fully conscious of the greatness of the Force within us. Every man is knowingly or unknowingly the instrument of a universal Power and, apart from the inner Presence, there is no such essential difference between one action and another, one kind of instrumentation and another as would warrant the folly of an egoistic pride. The difference between knowledge and ignorance is a grace of the Spirit; the breath of divine Power blows where it lists and fills today one and tomorrow another with the word or the puissance. If the potter shapes one pot more perfectly than another, the merit lies not in the vessel but the maker. The attitude of our mind must not be "This is my strength" or "Behold God's power in me", but rather "A Divine Power works in this mind and body and it is the same that works in all men and in the animal, in the plant and in the metal, in conscious and living things and in things apparently inconscient and inanimate."

This large view of the One working in all and of the whole world as the equal instrument of a divine action and gradual self-expression, if it becomes our entire experience, will help to eliminate all rajasic egoism out of us and even the sattwic ego-sense will begin to pass away from our nature.

The elimination of this form of ego leads straight towards the true instrumental action which is the essence of a perfect Karmayoga. For while we cherish the instrumental ego, we may pretend to ourselves that we are conscious instruments of the Divine, but in reality we are trying to make of the Divine Shakti an instrument of our own desires or our egoistic purpose. And even if the ego is subjected but not eliminated, we may indeed be engines of the Divine Work, but we shall be imperfect tools and deflect or impair the working by our mental errors, our vital distortions or the obstinate incapacities of our physical nature. If this ego disappears, then we can truly become, not only pure instruments consciously consenting to every turn of the divine Hand that moves us, but aware of our true nature, conscious portions of the one Eternal and Infinite put out in herself for her works by the supreme Shakti.

There is another greater step to be taken after the surrender of our instrumental ego to the Divine Shakti. It is not enough to know her as the one Cosmic Force that moves us and all creatures on the planes of mind, life and matter; for this is the lower Nature and, although the Divine Knowledge, Light, Power are there concealed and at work in this Ignorance and can break partly its veil and manifest something of their true character or descend from above and uplift these inferior workings, yet, even if we realise the One in a spiritualised mind, a spiritualised life-movement, a spiritualised body-consciousness, an imperfection remains in the dynamic parts. There is a stumbling response to the Supreme Power, a veil over the face of the Divine, a constant mixture of the Ignorance. It is only when we open to the Divine Shakti in the truth of her Force which transcends this lower Prakriti that we can be perfect instruments of her power and knowledge.

Not only liberation but perfection must be the aim of the Karmayoga. The Divine works through our nature and according to our nature; if our nature is imperfect, the work also will be imperfect, mixed, inadequate. Even it may be marred by gross errors, falsehoods, moral weaknesses, diverting influences. The work of the Divine will be done in us even then, but according to our weakness, not according to the strength and purity of its source. If ours were not an integral Yoga, if we sought only the liberation of the self within us or the motionless existence of Purusha separated from Prakriti, this dynamic imperfection might not matter. Calm, untroubled, not depressed, not elated, refusing to accept the perfection or imperfection, fault or merit, sin or virtue as ours, perceiving that it is the modes of Nature working in the field of her modes that make this mixture, we could withdraw into the silence of the spirit and, pure, untouched, witness only the workings of Prakriti. But in an integral realisation this can only be a step on the way, not our last resting-place. For we aim at the divine realisation not only in the immobility of the Spirit, but also in the movement of Nature. And this cannot be altogether until we can feel the presence and power of the Divine in every step, motion, figure of our activities, in every turn of our will, in every thought, feeling and impulse. No doubt, we can feel that in essence even in the nature of the Ignorance, but it is the divine Power and Presence in a disguise, a diminution, an inferior figure. Ours is a greater demand, that our nature shall be a power of the Divine in the Truth of the Divine, in the Light, in the force of the eternal self-conscient Will, in the wideness of the sempiternal Knowledge.

After the removal of the veil of ego, the removal of the veil of Nature and her inferior modes that govern our mind, life and body. As soon as the limits of the ego begin to fade, we see how that veil is constituted and detect the action of cosmic Nature in us, and in or behind cosmic Nature we sense the presence of the cosmic Self and the dynamis of the world-pervading Ishwara. The Master of the instrument stands behind all this working, and even within the working there is his touch and the drive of a great guiding or disposing Influence. It is no longer ego or ego-force that we serve; we obey the WorldMaster and his evolutionary impulse. At each step we can say in the language of the Sanskrit verse, "Even as I am appointed by Thee seated in my heart, so, O Lord, I act." But still this action may be of two very different kinds, one only illumined, the other transformed and uplifted into a greater supernature. For we may keep on in the way of action upheld and followed by our nature when by her and her illusion of egoism we were "turned as if mounted on a machine," but now with a perfect understanding of the mechanism and its utilisation for his world purposes by the Master of works whom we feel behind it. This is indeed as far as even many great Yogis have reached on the levels of spiritualised mind; but it need not be so always, for there is a greater supramental possibility. It is possible to rise beyond spiritualised mind and to act spontaneously in the living presence of the original divine Truth-Force of the Supreme Mother. Our motion one with her motion and merged in it, our will one with her will, our energy absolved in her energy, we shall feel her working through us as the Divine manifest in a supreme Wisdom-Power, and we shall be aware of the transformed mind, life and body only as the channels of a supreme Light and Force beyond them, infallible in its steps because transcendent and total in its knowledge. Of this Light and Force we shall not only be the recipients, channels, instruments, but become a part of it in a supreme uplifted abiding experience.

Already, before we reach this last perfection, we can have the union with the Divine in works in its extreme wideness, if not yet on its most luminous heights; for we perceive no longer merely Nature or the modes of Nature, but become conscious, in our physical movements, in our nervous and vital reactions, in our mental workings, of a Force greater than body, mind and life which takes hold of our limited instruments and drives all their motion. There is no longer the sense of ourselves moving, thinking or feeling but of that moving, feeling and thinking in us. This force that we feel is the universal Force of the Divine, which, veiled or unveiled, acting directly or permitting the use of its powers by beings in the cosmos, is the one Energy that alone exists and alone makes universal or individual action possible. For this force is the Divine itself in the body of its power; all is that, power of act, power of thought and knowledge, power of mastery and enjoyment, power of love. Conscious always and in everything, in ourselves and in others, of the Master of Works possessing, inhabiting, enjoying through this Force that is himself, becoming through it all existences and all happenings, we shall have arrived at the divine union through works and achieved by that fulfilment in works all that others have gained through absolute devotion or through pure knowledge. But there is still another step that calls us, an ascent out of this cosmic identity into the identity of the Divine Transcendence.

The Master of our works and our being is not merely a Godhead here within us, nor is he merely a cosmic Spirit or some kind of universal Power. The world and the Divine are not one and the same thing, as a certain kind of pantheistic thinking would like to believe. The world is an emanation; it depends upon something that manifests in it but is not limited by it: the Divine is not here alone; there is a Beyond, an eternal Transcendence. The individual being also in its spiritual part is not a formation in the cosmic existence—our ego, our mind, our life, our body are that; but the immutable spirit, the imperishable soul in us has come out of the Transcendence.

A Transcendent who is beyond all world and all Nature and yet possesses the world and its nature, who has descended with something of himself into it and is shaping it into that which as yet it is not, is the Source of our being, the Source of our works and their Master. But the seat of the Transcendent Consciousness is above in an absoluteness of divine Existence—and there too is the absolute Power, Truth, Bliss of the Eternal—of which our mentality can form no conception and of which even our greatest spiritual experience is only a diminished reflection in the spiritualised mind and heart, a faint shadow, a thin derivate. Yet proceeding from it there is a sort of golden corona of Light, Power, Bliss and Truth—a divine Truth-

Consciousness as the ancient mystics called it, a Supermind, a Gnosis, with which this world of a lesser consciousness proceeding by Ignorance is in secret relation and which alone maintains it and prevents it from falling into a disintegrated chaos. The powers we are now satisfied to call gnosis, intuition or illumination are only fainter lights of which that is the full and flaming source, and between the highest human intelligence and it there lie many levels of ascending consciousness, highest mental or overmental, which we would have to conquer before we arrived there or could bring down its greatness and glory here. Yet, however difficult, that ascent, that victory is the destiny of the human spirit and that luminous descent or bringing down of the divine Truth is the inevitable term of the troubled evolution of the earth-nature; that intended consummation is its *raison d'être*, our culminating state and the explanation of our terrestrial existence. For though the transcendental Divine is already here as the Purushottama in the secret heart of our mystery, he is veiled by many coats and disguises of his magic world-wide Yoga-Maya; it is only by the ascent and victory of the Soul here in the body that the disguises can fall away and the dynamis of the supreme Truth replace this tangled weft of half-truth that becomes creative error, this emergent Knowledge that is converted by its plunge into the inconscience of Matter and its slow partial return towards itself into an effective Ignorance.

For here in the world, though the Gnosis is there secretly behind existence, what acts is not the Gnosis but a magic of Knowledge-Ignorance, an incalculable yet apparently mechanical Overmind Maya. The Divine appears to us here in one view as an equal, inactive and impersonal Witness Spirit, an immobile consenting Purusha not bound by quality or Space or Time, whose support or sanction is given impartially to the play of all action and energies which the transcendent Will has once permitted and authorised to fulfil themselves in the cosmos. This Witness Spirit, this immobile Self in things, seems to will nothing and determine nothing; yet we become aware that his very passivity, his silent presence compels all things to travel even in their ignorance towards a divine goal and attracts through division towards a yet unrealised oneness. Yet no supreme infallible Divine Will seems to be there, only a widely deployed Cosmic Energy or a mechanical executive Process, Prakriti. This is one side of the cosmic Self; the other presents itself as a universal Divine, one in being, multiple in personality and power, who conveys to us, when we enter into the consciousness of his universal forces, a sense of infinite quality and will and act and worldwide knowledge and a one yet innumerable delight; for through him we become one with all existences not only in their essence but in their play of action, see ourself in all and all in ourself, perceive all knowledge and thought and feeling as motions of the one Mind and Heart, all energy and action as kinetics of the one Will in power, all Matter and form as particles of the one Body, all personalities as projections of the one

Person, all egos as deformations of the one and sole real "I" in existence. In him we no longer stand separate, but lose our active ego in the universal movement, even as by the Witness who is without qualities and for ever unattached and unentangled, we lose our static ego in the universal peace.

And yet there remains a contradiction between these two terms, the aloof divine Silence and the all-embracing divine Action, which we may heal in ourselves in a certain manner, in a certain high degree which seems to us complete, yet is not complete because it cannot altogether transform and conquer. A universal Peace, Light, Power, Bliss is ours, but its effective expression is not that of the Truth-Consciousness, the divine Gnosis, but still, though wonderfully freed, uplifted and illumined, supports only the present self-expression of the Cosmic Spirit and does not transform, as would a transcendental Descent, the ambiguous symbols and veiled mysteries of a world of Ignorance. Ourselves are free, but the earth-consciousness remains in bondage; only a further transcendental ascent and descent can entirely heal the contradiction and transform and deliver.

For there is yet a third intensely close and personal aspect of the Master of Works which is a key to his sublimest hidden mystery and ecstasy; for he detaches from the secret of the hidden Transcendence and the ambiguous display of the cosmic Movement an individual Power of the Divine that can mediate between the two and bridge our passage from the one to the other. In this aspect the transcendent and universal person of the Divine conforms itself to our individualised personality and accepts a personal relation with us, at once identified with us as our supreme Self and yet close and different as our Master, Friend, Lover, Teacher, our Father and our Mother, our Playmate in the great world-game who has disguised himself throughout as friend and enemy, helper and opponent and, in all relations and in all workings that affect us, has led our steps towards our perfection and our release. It is through this more personal manifestation that we are admitted to some possibility of the complete transcendental experience; for in him we meet the One not merely in a liberated calm and peace, not merely with a passive or active submission in our works or through the mystery of union with a universal Knowledge and Power filling and guiding us, but with an ecstasy of divine Love and divine Delight that shoots up beyond silent Witness and active World-Power to some positive divination of a greater beatific secret. For it is not so much knowledge leading to some ineffable Absolute, not so much works lifting us beyond world-process to the originating supreme Knower and Master, but rather this thing most intimate to us, yet at present most obscure, which keeps for us wrapped in its passionate veil the deep and rapturous secret of the transcendent Godhead and some absolute positiveness of its perfect Being, its all-concentrating Bliss, its mystic Ananda.

But the individual relation with the Divine does not always or from the beginning bring into force a widest enlargement or a highest self-exceeding. At first this Godhead close to our being or immanent within us can be felt fully only in the scope of our personal nature and experience, a Leader and Master, a Guide and Teacher, a Friend and Lover, or else a spirit, power or presence, constituting and uplifting our upward and enlarging movement by the force of his intimate reality inhabiting the heart or presiding over our nature from above even our highest intelligence. It is our personal evolution that is his preoccupation, a personal relation with him that his our joy and fulfilment, the building of our nature into his divine image that is our selffinding and perfection. The outside world seems to exist only as a field for this growth and a provider of materials or of helping and opposing forces for its successive stages. Our works done in that world are his works, but even when they serve some temporary universal end, their main purpose for us is to make outwardly dynamic or give inward power to our relations with this immanent Divine. Many seekers ask for no more or see the continuation and fulfilment of this spiritual flowering only in heavens beyond; the union is consummated and made perpetual in an eternal dwelling-place of his perfection, joy and beauty. But this is not enough for the integral seeker; however intense and beautiful, a personal isolated achievement cannot be his sole aim or his entire experience. A time must come when the personal opens out into the universal; our very individuality, spiritual, mental, vital, physical even, becomes universalised: it is seen as a power of his universal force and cosmic spirit, or else it contains the universe in that ineffable wideness which comes to the individual consciousness when it breaks its bonds and flows upward towards the Transcendent and on every side into the Infinite.

In a Yoga lived entirely on the spiritualised mental plane it is possible and even usual for these three fundamental aspects of the Divine—the Individual or Immanent, the Cosmic and the Transcendent—to stand out as separate realisations. Each by itself then appears sufficient to satisfy the yearning of the seeker. Alone with the personal Divine in the inner heart's illumined secret chamber, he can build his being into the Beloved's image and ascend out of fallen Nature to dwell with him in some heaven of the Spirit. Absolved in the cosmic wideness, released from ego, his personality reduced to a point of working of the universal Force, himself calm, liberated, deathless in universality, motionless in the Witness Self even while outspread without limit in unending Space and Time, he can enjoy in the world the freedom of the Timeless. One-pointed towards some ineffable Transcendence, casting away his personality, shedding from him the labour and trouble of the universal Dynamis, he can escape into an inexpressible Nirvana, annul all things in an intolerant exaltation of flight into the Incommunicable.

But none of these achievements is enough for one who seeks the wide completeness of an integral Yoga. An individual salvation is not enough for him; for he finds himself opening to a cosmic consciousness which far exceeds by its breadth and vastness the narrower intensity of a limited individual fulfilment, and its call is imperative; driven by that immense compulsion, he must break through all separative boundaries, spread himself in world-Nature, contain the universe. Above too, there is urgent upon him a dynamic realisation pressing from the Supreme upon this world of beings, and only some encompassing and exceeding of the cosmic consciousness can release into manifestation here that yet unlavished splendour. But the cosmic consciousness too is not sufficient; for it is not all the Divine Reality, not integral. There is a divine secret behind personality that he must discover; there, waiting in it to be delivered here into Time, stands the mystery of the embodiment of the Transcendence. In the cosmic consciousness there remains at the end a hiatus, an unequal equation of a highest Knowledge that can liberate but not effectuate with a Power seeming to use a limited Knowledge or masking itself with a surface Ignorance that can create but creates imperfection or a perfection transient, limited and in fetters. On one side there is a free undynamic Witness and on the other side a bound Executrix of action who has not been given all the means of action. The reconciliation of these companions and opposites seems to be reserved, postponed, held back in an Unmanifest still beyond us. But, again, a mere escape into some absolute Transcendence leaves personality unfulfilled and the universal action inconclusive and cannot satisfy the integral seeker. He feels that the Truth that is for ever is a Power that creates as well as a stable Existence; it is not a Power solely of illusory or ignorant manifestation. The eternal Truth can manifest its truths in Time; it can create in Knowledge and not only in Inconscience and Ignorance. A divine Descent no less than an ascent to the Divine is possible; there is a prospect of the bringing down of a future perfection and a present deliverance. As his knowledge widens, it becomes for him more and more evident that it was this for which the Master of Works cast down the soul within him here as a spark of his fire into the darkness, that it might grow there into a centre of the Light that is for ever.

The Transcendent, the Universal, the Individual are three powers overarching, underlying and penetrating the whole manifestation; this is the first of the Trinities. In the unfolding of consciousness also, these are the three fundamental terms and none of them can be neglected if we would have the experience of the whole Truth of existence. Out of the individual we wake into a vaster freer cosmic consciousness; but out of the universal too with its complex of forms and powers we must emerge by a still greater self-exceeding into a consciousness without limits that is founded on the Absolute. And yet in this ascension we do not really abolish but take up and transfigure what we seem to leave; for there is a height where the three live eternally in each other, on that height they are blissfully joined in a nodus of their harmonised oneness. But that summit is above the highest and largest spiritualised mentality, even if some reflection of it can be experienced there; mind, to attain to it, to live there, must exceed itself and be transformed into a supramental gnostic light, power and substance. In this lower diminished consciousness a harmony can indeed be attempted, but it must always remain imperfect; a coordination is possible, not a simultaneous fused fulfilment. An ascent out of the mind is, for any greater realisation, imperative. Or else, there must be, with the ascent or consequent to it, a dynamic descent of the self-existent Truth that exists always uplifted in its own light above Mind, eternal, prior to the manifestation of Life and Matter.

For Mind is Maya, *sat-asat*: there is a field of embrace of the true and the false, the existent and the non-existent, and it is in that ambiguous field that Mind seems to reign; but even in its own reign it is in truth a diminished consciousness, it is not part of the original and supremely originating power of the Eternal. Even if Mind is able to reflect some image of essential Truth in its substance, yet the dynamic force and action of Truth appears in it always broken and divided. All Mind can do is to piece together the fragments or deduce a unity; truth of Mind is only a half-truth or a portion of a puzzle. Mental knowledge is always relative, partial and inconclusive, and its outgoing action and creation come out still more confused in its steps or precise only in narrow limits and by imperfect piecings together. Even in this diminished consciousness the Divine manifests as a Spirit in Mind, just as he moves as a Spirit in Life or dwells still more obscurely as a Spirit in Matter; but not here is his full dynamic revelation, not here the perfect identities of the Eternal. Only when we cross the border into a larger luminous consciousness and self-aware substance where divine Truth is a native and not a stranger, will there be revealed to us the Master of our existence in the imperishable integral truth of his being and his powers and his workings. Only there, too, will his works in us assume the flawless movement of his unfailing supramental purpose.

∽

But that is the end of a long and difficult journey, and the Master of works does not wait till then to meet the seeker on the path of Yoga and put his secret or half-shown Hand upon him and upon his life and actions. Already he was there in the world as the Originator and Receiver of works behind the dense veils of the Inconscient, disguised in force of Life, visible to the Mind through symbol godheads and figures. It may well be in these disguises that he first meets the soul destined to the way of the integral

Yoga. Or even, wearing still vaguer masks, he may be conceived by us as an Ideal or mentalised as an abstract Power of Love, Good, Beauty or Knowledge; or, as we turn our feet towards the Way, he may come to us veiled as the call of Humanity or a Will in things that drives towards the deliverance of the world from the grasp of Darkness and Falsehood and Death and Suffering—the great quaternary of the Ignorance. Then, after we have entered the path, he envelops us with his wide and mighty liberating Impersonality or moves near to us with the face and form of a personal Godhead. In and around us we feel a Power that upholds and protects and cherishes; we hear a Voice that guides; a conscious Will greater than ourselves rules us; an imperative Force moves our thought and actions and our very body; an ever-widening Consciousness assimilates ours, a living Light of Knowledge lights all within, or a Beatitude invades us; a Mightiness presses from above, concrete, massive and overpowering, and penetrates and pours itself into the very stuff of our nature; a Peace sits there, a Light, a Bliss, a Strength, a Greatness. Or there are relations, personal, intimate as life itself, sweet as love, encompassing like the sky, deep like deep waters. A Friend walks at our side; a Lover is with us in our heart's secrecy; a Master of the Work and the Ordeal points our way; a Creator of things uses us as his instrument; we are in the arms of the eternal Mother. All these more seizable aspects in which the Ineffable meets us are truths and not mere helpful symbols or useful imaginations; but as we progress, their first imperfect formulations in our experience yield to a larger vision of the one Truth that is behind them. At each step their mere mental masks are shed and they acquire a larger, a profounder, a more intimate significance. At last on the supramental borders all these Godheads combine their forces and, without at all ceasing to be, coalesce together. On this path the Divine Aspects are not revealed in order to be cast away; they are not temporary spiritual conveniences or compromises with an illusory Consciousness or dream-figures mysteriously cast upon us by the incommunicable superconscience of the Absolute; on the contrary, their power increases and their absoluteness reveals itself as they draw near to the Truth from which they issue.

For that now superconscient Transcendence is a Power as well as an Existence. The supramental Transcendence is not a vacant Wonder, but an Inexpressible which contains for ever all essential things that have issued from it; it holds them there in their supreme everlasting reality and their own characteristic absolutes. The diminution, division, degradation that create here the sense of an unsatisfactory puzzle, a mystery of Maya, themselves diminish and fall from us in our ascension, and the Divine Powers assume their real forms and appear more and more as the terms of a Truth in process of realisation here. A soul of the Divine is here slowly awaking out of its involution and concealment in the material Inconscience. The Master of our works is not a Master of illusions, but a supreme Reality who is working out his self-expressive realities delivered slowly from the cocoons of the Ignorance in which for the purposes of an evolutionary manifestation they were allowed for a while to slumber. For the supramental Transcendence is not a thing absolutely apart and unconnected with our present existence. It is a greater Light out of which all this has come for the adventure of the Soul lapsing into the Inconscience and emerging out of it, and, while that adventure proceeds, it waits superconscient above our minds till it can become conscious in us. Hereafter it will unveil itself and by the unveiling reveal to us all the significance of our own being and our works; for it will disclose the Divine whose fuller manifestation in the world will release and accomplish that covert significance.

In that disclosure the Transcendent Divine will be more and more made known to us as the Supreme Existence and the Perfect Source of all that we are; but equally we shall see him as a Master of works and creation prepared to pour out more and more of himself into the field of his manifestation. The cosmic consciousness and its action will appear no longer as a huge regulated Chance, but as a field of the manifestation; there the Divine is seen as a presiding and pervading Cosmic Spirit who receives all out of the Transcendence and develops what descends into forms that are now an opaque disguise or a baffling half-disguise, but destined to be a transparent revelation. The individual consciousness will recover its true sense and action; for it is the form of a Soul sent out from the Supreme and, in spite of all appearances, a nucleus or nebula in which the Divine Mother-Force is at work for the victorious embodiment of the timeless and formless Divine in Time and Matter. This will reveal itself slowly to our vision and experience as the will of the Master of works and as their own ultimate significance, which alone gives to world-creation and to our own action in the world a light and a meaning. To recognise that and to strive towards its effectuation is the whole burden of the Way of Divine Works in the integral Yoga.

CHAPTER XII. THE DIVINE WORK

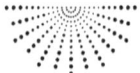

ONE QUESTION remains for the seeker upon the way of works, when his quest is or seems to have come to its natural end,—whether any work or what work is left for the soul after liberation and to what purpose? Equality has been seated in the nature or governs the whole nature; there has been achieved a radical deliverance from the ego-idea, from the pervading ego-sense, from all feelings and impulsions of the ego and its self-will and desires. The entire self-consecration has been made not only in thought and heart but in all the complexities of the being. A complete purity or transcendence of the three gunas has been harmoniously established. The soul has seen the Master of its works and lives in his presence or is consciously contained in his being or is unified with him or feels him in the heart or above and obeys his dictates. It has known its true being and cast away the veil of the Ignorance. What work then remains for the worker in man and with what motive, to what end, in what spirit will it be done?

There is one answer with which we are very familiar in India; no work at all remains, for the rest is quiescence. When the soul can live in the eternal presence of the Supreme or when it is unified with the Absolute, the object of our existence in the world, if it can be said to have an object, at once ceases. Man, released from the curse of self-division and the curse of Ignorance, is released too from that other affliction, the curse of works. All action would then be a derogation from the supreme state and a return into the Ignorance. This attitude towards life is supported by an idea founded on the error of the vital nature to which action is dictated only by one or all of three inferior motives, necessity, restless instinct and impulse or desire. The instinct or impulse quiescent, desire extinguished, what place is there for works? Some mechanical necessity might remain but no other, and even that would cease for ever with the fall of the body. But after all, even so, while life remains, action is unavoidable. Mere thinking or, in the absence of thought, mere living is itself an act and a cause of many effects. All existence in the world is work, force, potency, and has a dynamic effect in the whole by its mere presence, even the inertia of the clod, even the silence of the immobile Buddha on the verge of Nirvana. There is the question only of the manner of the action, the instruments that are used or that act of themselves, and the spirit and knowledge of the worker. For in reality, no man works, but Nature works through him for the self-expression of a Power within that proceeds from the Infinite. To know that and live in the presence and in the being of the Master of Nature, free from desire and the illusion of personal impulsion, is the one thing needful. That and not the bodily cessation of action is the true release; for the bondage of works at once ceases. A man might sit still and motionless for ever and yet be as much bound to the Ignorance as the animal or the insect. But if he can make this greater consciousness dynamic within him, then all the work of all the worlds could pass through him and yet he would remain at rest, absolute in calm and peace, free from all bondage. Action in the world is given us first as a means for our self-development and self-fulfilment; but even if we reached a last possible divine self-completeness, it would still remain as a means for the fulfilment of the divine intention in the world and of the larger universal self of which each being is a portion—a portion that has come down with it from the Transcendence.

In a certain sense, when his Yoga has reached a certain culmination, works cease for a man; for he has no further personal necessity of works, no sense of works being done by him; but there is no need to flee from action or to take refuge in a blissful inertia. For now he acts as the Divine Existence acts without any binding necessity and without any compelling ignorance. Even in doing works *he* does not work at all; he undertakes no personal initiative. It is the Divine Shakti that works in him through his nature; his action develops through the spontaneity of a supreme Force by which his instruments are possessed, of which he is a part, with whose will his will is identical and his power is her power. The spirit within him contains, supports and watches this action; it presides over it in knowledge but is not glued or clamped to the work by attachment or need, is not bound by desire of its fruit, is not enslaved to any movement or impulse.

It is a common error to suppose that action is impossible or at least meaningless without desire. If desire ceases, we are told, action also must cease. But this, like other too simply comprehensive generalisations, is more attractive to the cutting and defining mind than true. The major part of the work done in the universe is accomplished without any interference of desire; it proceeds by the calm necessity and spontaneous law of Nature. Even man constantly does work of various kinds by a spontaneous impulse, intuition, instinct or acts in obedience to a natural necessity and law of forces without either mental planning or the urge of a conscious vital volition or emotional desire. Often enough his act is contrary to his intention or his desire; it proceeds out of him in subjection to a need or compulsion, in submission to an impulse, in obedience to a force in him that pushes for self-expression or in conscious pursuance of a higher principle. Desire is an additional lure to which Nature has given a great part in the life of animated beings in order to produce a certain kind of rajasic action necessary for her intermediate ends; but it is not her sole or even her chief engine. It has its great use while it endures: it helps us to rise out of inertia, it contradicts many tamasic forces which would otherwise inhibit action. But the seeker who has advanced far on the way of works has passed beyond this intermediate stage in which desire is a helpful engine. Its push is no longer indispensable for his action, but is rather a terrible hindrance and source of stumbling, inefficiency and failure. Others are obliged to obey a personal choice or motive, but he has to learn to act with an impersonal or a universal mind or as a part or an instrument of an infinite Person. A calm indifference, a joyful impartiality or a blissful response to a divine Force, whatever its dictate, is the condition of his doing any effective work or undertaking any worth-while action. Not desire, not attachment must drive him, but a Will that stirs in a divine peace, a Knowledge that moves from the transcendent Light, a glad Impulse that is a force from the supreme Ananda.

In an advanced stage of the Yoga it is indifferent to the seeker, in the sense of any personal preference, what action he shall do or not do; even whether he shall act or not, is not decided by his personal choice or pleasure. Always he is moved to do whatever is in consonance with the Truth or whatever the Divine demands through his nature. A false conclusion is sometimes drawn from this that the spiritual man, accepting the position in which Fate or God or his past Karma has placed him, content to work in the field and cadre of the family, clan, caste, nation, occupation which are his by birth and circumstance, will not and even perhaps ought not to make any movement to exceed them or to pursue any great mundane end. Since he has really no work to do, since he has only to use works, no matter what works, as long as he is in the body in order to arrive at liberation or, having arrived, only to obey the supreme Will and do whatever it dictates, the actual field given him is sufficient for the purpose. Once free, he has only to continue working in the sphere assigned to him by Fate and circumstances till the great hour arrives when he can at last disappear into the Infinite. To insist on any particular end or to work for some great mundane object is to fall into the illusion of works; it is to entertain the error that terrestrial life has an intelligible intention and contains objects worthy of pursuit. The great theory of Illusion, which is a practical denial of the Divine in the world, even when in idea it acknowledges the Presence, is once more before us. But the Divine is here in the world,—not only in status but in dynamis, not only as a spiritual self and presence but as power, force, energy,—and therefore a divine work in the world is possible.

There is no narrow principle, no field of cabined action that can be imposed on the Karmayogin as his rule or his province. This much is true that every kind of works, whether small to man's imagination or great, petty in scope or wide, can be equally used in the progress towards liberation or for self-discipline. This much is also true that after liberation a man may dwell in any sphere of life and in any kind of action and fulfil there his existence in the Divine. According as he is moved by the Spirit, he may remain in the sphere assigned to him by birth and circumstances or break that framework and go forth to an untrammelled action which shall be the fitting body of his greatened consciousness and higher knowledge. To the outward eyes of men the inner liberation may make no apparent difference in his outward acts; or, on the contrary, the freedom and infinity within may translate itself into an outward dynamic working so large and new that all regards are drawn by this novel force. If such be the intention of the Supreme within him, the liberated soul may be content with a subtle and limited action within the old human surroundings which will in no way seek to change their outward appearance. But it may too be called to a work which will not only alter the forms and sphere of its own external life but, leaving nothing around it unchanged or unaffected, create a new world or a new order.

∽

A prevalent idea would persuade us that the sole aim of liberation is to secure for the individual soul freedom from physical rebirth in the unstable life of the universe. If this freedom is once assured, there is no further work for it in life here or elsewhere or only that which the continued existence of the body demands or the unfulfilled effects of past lives necessitate. This little, rapidly exhausted or consumed by the fire of Yoga, will cease with the departure of the released soul from the body. The aim of escape from rebirth, now long fixed in the Indian mentality as the highest object of the soul, has replaced the enjoyment of a heaven beyond fixed in the mentality of the devout by many religions as their divine lure.

Indian religion also upheld that earlier and lower call when the gross external interpretation of the Vedic hymns was the dominant creed, and the dualists in later India also have kept that as part of their supreme spiritual motive. Undoubtedly a release from the limitations of the mind and body into an eternal peace, rest, silence of the Spirit, makes a higher appeal than the offer of a heaven of mental joys or eternised physical pleasures, but this too after all is a lure; its insistence on the mind's world-weariness, the life-being's shrinking from the adventure of birth, strikes a chord of weakness and cannot be the supreme motive. The desire of personal salvation, however high its form, is an outcome of ego; it rests on the idea of our own individuality and its desire for its personal good or welfare, its longing for a release from suffering or its cry for the extinction of the trouble of becoming and makes that the supreme aim of our existence. To rise beyond the desire of personal salvation is necessary for the complete rejection of this basis of ego. If we seek the Divine, it should be for the sake of the Divine and for nothing else, because that is the supreme call of our being, the deepest truth of the spirit. The pursuit of liberation, of the soul's freedom, of the realisation of our true and highest self, of union with the Divine, is justified only because it is the highest law of our nature, because it is the attraction of that which is lower in us to that which is highest, because it is the Divine Will in us. That is its sufficient justification and its one truest reason; all other motives are excrescences, minor or incidental truths or useful lures which the soul must abandon, the moment their utility has passed and the state of oneness with the Supreme and with all beings has become our normal consciousness and the bliss of that state our spiritual atmosphere.

    Often, we see this desire of personal salvation overcome by another attraction which also belongs to the higher turn of our nature and which indicates the essential character of the action the liberated soul must pursue. It is that which is implied in the great legend of the Amitabha Buddha who turned away when his spirit was on the threshold of Nirvana and took the vow never to cross it while a single being remained in the sorrow and the Ignorance. It is that which underlies the sublime verse of the Bhagavata Purana, "I desire not the supreme state with all its eight siddhis nor the cessation of rebirth; may I assume the sorrow of all creatures who suffer and enter into them so that they may be made free from grief." It is that which inspires a remarkable passage in a letter of Swami Vivekananda. "I have lost all wish for my salvation," wrote the great Vedantin, "may I be born again and again and suffer thousands of miseries so that I may worship the only God that exists, the only God I believe in, the sum-total of all souls,—and above all, my God the wicked, my God the miserable, my God the poor of all races, of all species is the special object of my worship. He who is the high and low, the saint and the sinner, the god and the worm, Him worship, the visible, the knowable, the real, the omnipresent; break all other idols. In whom there is neither past life nor future birth, nor death nor going nor coming, in whom we always have been and always will be one, Him worship; break all other idols."

The last two sentences contain indeed the whole gist of the matter. The true salvation or the true freedom from the chain of rebirth is not the rejection of terrestrial life or the individual's escape by a spiritual self-annihilation, even as the true renunciation is not the mere physical abandonment of family and society; it is the inner identification with the Divine in whom there is no limitation of past life and future birth but instead the eternal existence of the unborn Soul. He who is free inwardly, even doing actions, does nothing at all, says the Gita; for it is Nature that works in him under the control of the Lord of Nature. Equally, even if he assumes a hundred times the body, he is free from any chain of birth or mechanical wheel of existence since he lives in the unborn and undying spirit and not in the life of the body. Therefore attachment to the escape from rebirth is one of the idols which, whoever keeps, the sadhaka of the integral Yoga must break and cast away from him. For his Yoga is not limited to the realisation of the Transcendent beyond all world by the individual soul; it embraces also the realisation of the Universal, "the sum-total of all souls", and cannot therefore be confined to the movement of a personal salvation and escape.

Even in his transcendence of cosmic limitations he is still one with all in God; a divine work remains for him in the universe.

That work cannot be fixed by any mind-made rule or human standard; for his consciousness has moved away from human law and limits and passed into the divine liberty, away from government by the external and transient into the self-rule of the inner and eternal, away from the binding forms of the finite into the free self-determination of the Infinite. "Howsoever he lives and acts," says the Gita, "he lives and acts in Me." The rules which the intellect of men lays down cannot apply to the liberated soul,— by the external criteria and tests which their mental associations and prejudgments prescribe, such a one cannot be judged; he is outside the narrow jurisdiction of these fallible tribunals. It is immaterial whether he wears the garb of the ascetic or lives the full life of the householder; whether he spends his days in what men call holy works or in the many-sided activities of the world; whether he devotes himself to the direct leading of men to the Light like Buddha, Christ or Shankara or governs kingdoms like Janaka or stands before men like Sri Krishna as a politician or a leader of armies; what he eats or drinks; what are his habits or his pursuits; whether he fails or succeeds; whether his work be one of construction or of destruction; whether he supports or restores an old order or labours to replace it by a new; whether his associates are those whom men delight to honour or those whom their sense of superior righteousness outcastes and reprobates; whether his life and deeds are approved by his contemporaries or he is condemned as a misleader of men and a fomenter of religious, moral or social heresies. He is not governed by the judgments of men or the laws laid down by the ignorant; he obeys an inner voice and is moved by an unseen Power. His real life is within and this is its description that he lives, moves and acts in God, in the Divine, in the Infinite.

But if his action is governed by no external rule, one rule it will observe that is not external; it will be dictated by no personal desire or aim, but will be a part of a conscious and eventually a well-ordered because self-ordered divine working in the world. The Gita declares that the action of the liberated man must be directed not by desire, but towards the keeping together of the world, its government, guidance, impulsion, maintenance in the path appointed to it. This injunction has been interpreted in the sense that the world being an illusion in which most men must be kept, since they are unfit for liberation, he must so act outwardly as to cherish in them an attachment to their customary works laid down for them by the social law. If so, it would be a poor and petty rule and every noble heart would reject it to follow rather the divine vow of Amitabha Buddha, the sublime prayer of the Bhagavata, the passionate aspiration of Vivekananda. But if we accept rather the view that the world is a divinely guided movement of Nature emerging in man towards God and that this is the work in which the Lord of the Gita declares that he is ever occupied although he himself has nothing ungained that he has yet to win, then a deep and true sense will appear for this great injunction. To participate in that divine work, to live for God in the world will be the rule of the Karmayogin; to live for God in the world and therefore so to act that the Divine may more and more manifest himself and the world go forward by whatever way of its obscure pilgrimage and move nearer to the divine ideal.

How he shall do this, in what particular way, can be decided by no general rule. It must develop or define itself from within; the decision lies between God and our self, the Supreme Self and the individual self that is the instrument of the work; even before liberation, it is from the inner self, as soon as we become conscious of it, that there rises the sanction, the spiritually determined choice. It is altogether from within that must come the knowledge of the work that has to be done. There is no particular work, no law or form or outwardly fixed or invariable way of works which can be said to be that of the liberated being. The phrase used in the Gita to express this work that has to be done has indeed been interpreted in the sense that we must do our duty without regard to the fruit. But this is a conception born of European culture which is ethical rather than spiritual and external rather than inwardly profound in its concepts. No such general thing as duty exists; we have only duties, often in conflict with each other, and these are determined by our environment, our social relations, our external status in life. They are of great value in training the immature moral nature and setting up a standard which discourages the action of selfish desire. It has already been said that so long as the seeker has no inner light, he must govern himself by the best light he has, and duty, a principle, a cause are among the standards he may temporarily erect and observe. But for all that, duties are external things, not stuff of the soul and cannot be the ultimate standard of action in this path. It is the duty of the soldier to fight when called upon, even to fire upon his own kith and kin; but such a standard or any akin to it cannot be imposed on the liberated man. On the other hand, to love or have compassion, to obey the highest truth of our being, to follow the command of the Divine are not duties; these things are a law of the nature as it rises towards the Divine, an outflowing of action from a soul-state, a high reality of the spirit. The action of the liberated doer of works must be even such an outflowing from the soul; it must come to him or out of him as a natural result of his spiritual union with the Divine and not be formed by an edifying construction of the mental thought and will, the practical reason or the social sense. In the ordinary life a personal, social or traditional constructed rule, standard or ideal is the guide; once the spiritual journey has begun, this must be replaced by an inner and outer rule or way of living necessary for our self-discipline, liberation and perfection, a way of living proper to the path we follow or enjoined by the spiritual guide and master, the Guru, or else dictated by a Guide within us. But in the last state of the soul's infinity and freedom all outward standards are replaced or laid aside and there is left only a spontaneous and integral obedience to the Divine with whom we are in union and an action spontaneously fulfilling the integral spiritual truth of our being and nature.

It is this deeper sense in which we must accept the dictum of the Gita that action determined and governed by the nature must be our law of works. It is not, certainly, the superficial temperament or the character or habitual impulses that are meant, but in the literal sense of the Sanskrit word our "own being", our essential nature, the divine stuff of our souls. Whatever springs from this root or flows from these sources is profound, essential, right; the rest—opinions, impulses, habits, desires—may be merely surface formations or casual vagaries of the being or impositions from outside. They shift and change, but this remains constant. It is not the executive forms taken by Nature in us that are ourselves or the abidingly constant and expressive shape of ourselves; it is the spiritual being in us—and this includes the soul-becoming of it—that persists through time in the universe.

We cannot, however, easily distinguish this true inner law of our being; it is kept screened from us so long as the heart and intellect remain unpurified from egoism: till then we follow superficial and impermanent ideas, impulses, desires, suggestions and impositions of all kinds from our environment or work out formations of our temporary mental, vital, physical personality—that passing experimental and structural self which has been made for us by an interaction between our being and the pressure of a lower cosmic Nature. In proportion as we are purified, the true being within declares itself more clearly; our will is less entangled in suggestions from outside or shut up in our own superficial mental constructions. Egoism renounced, the nature purified, action will come from the soul's dictates, from the depths or the heights of the spirit, or it will be openly governed by the Lord who was all the time seated secretly within our heart. The supreme and final word of the Gita for the Yogin is that he should leave all conventional formulas of belief and action, all fixed and external rules of conduct, all constructions of the outward or surface Nature, *dharmas*, and take refuge in the Divine alone. Free from desire and attachment, one with all beings, living in the infinite Truth and Purity and acting out of the profoundest deeps of his inner consciousness, governed by his immortal, divine and highest Self, all his works will be directed by the Power within through that essential spirit and nature in us which, knowing, warring, working, loving, serving, is always divine, towards the fulfilment of God in the world, an expression of the Eternal in Time.

A divine action arising spontaneously, freely, infallibly from the light and force of our spiritual self in union with the Divine is the last state of this integral Yoga of Works. The truest reason why we must seek liberation is not to be delivered, individually, from the sorrow of the world, though that deliverance too will be given to us, but that we may be one with the Divine, the Supreme, the Eternal. The truest reason why we must seek perfection, a supreme status, purity, knowledge, strength, love, capacity, is not that personally we may enjoy the divine Nature or be even as the gods, though that enjoyment too will be ours, but because this liberation and perfection are the divine Will in us, the highest truth of our self in Nature, the always intended goal of a progressive manifestation in the universe. The divine Nature, free and perfect and blissful, must be manifested in the individual in order that it may manifest in the world. Even in the Ignorance the individual lives really in the universal and for the universal Purpose, for in the very act of pursuing the purposes and desires of his ego, he is forced by Nature to contribute by his egoistic action to her work and purpose in the worlds; but it is without conscious intention, imperfectly done, and his contribution is to her half-evolved and half-conscient, her imperfect and crude movement. To escape from ego and be united with the Divine is at once the liberation and the consummation of his individuality; so liberated, purified, perfected, the individual—the divine soul—lives consciously and entirely, as was from the first intended, in and for the cosmic and transcendent Divine and for his Will in the universe.

In the Way of Knowledge we may arrive at a point where we can leap out of personality and universe, escape from all thought and will and works and all way of Nature and, absorbed and taken up into Eternity, plunge into the Transcendence; that, though not obligatory on the God-knower, may be the soul's decision, the turn pursued by the self within us. In the Way of Devotion we may reach through an intensity of adoration and joy union with the supreme All-Beloved and remain eternally in the ecstasy of his presence, absorbed in him alone, intimately in one world of bliss with him; that then may be our being's impulsion, its spiritual choice. But in the Way of Works another prospect opens; for travelling on that path, we can enter into liberation and perfection by becoming of one law and power of nature with the Eternal; we are identified with him in our will and dynamic self as much as in our spiritual status; a divine way of works is the natural outcome of this union, a divine living in a spiritual freedom the body of its self-expression. In the Integral Yoga these three lines of approach give up their exclusions, meet and coalesce or spring out of each other; liberated from the mind's veil over the self, we live in the Transcendence, enter by the adoration of the heart into the oneness of a supreme love and bliss, and all our forces of being uplifted into the one Force, our will and works surrendered into the one Will and Power, assume the dynamic perfection of the divine Nature.

ALSO BY SRI AUROBINDO

ESSAYS ON THE GITA

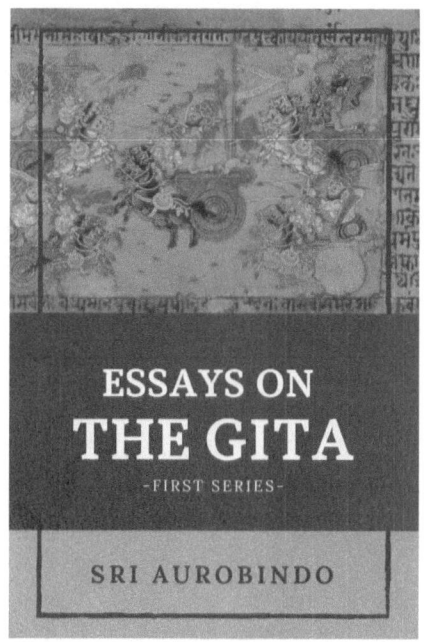

FIRST SERIES

- ISBN PAPERBACK: 9782357286313
- ISBN HARDCOVER: 9782357286320
- ISBN E-BOOK: 9782357286337

SECOND SERIES

- ISBN PAPERBACK: 9782357286481
- ISBN HARDCOVER: 9782357286498
- ISBN E-BOOK: 9782357286504

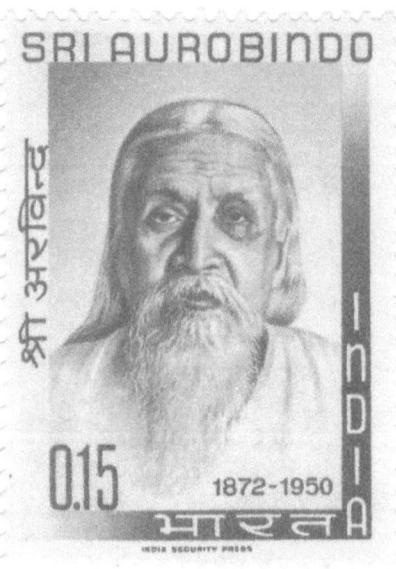

Copyright © 2020 by ALICIA EDITIONS
Credits: Canva
All rights reserved.
No part of this book may be reproduced in any form or by any electronic or mechanical means, including information storage and retrieval systems, without written permission from the author, except for the use of brief quotations in a book review.